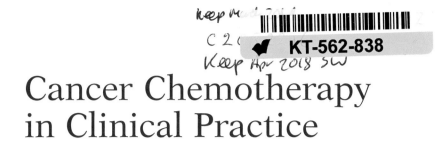

Cancer Chemotherapy in Clinical Practice

Terry Priestman

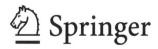 Springer

Terry Priestman, MD, FRCP, FRCR
New Cross Hospital
Wolverhampton
UK

British Library Cataloguing in Publication Data
Priestman, Terry J.
    Cancer chemotherapy in clinical practice
    1. Cancer - Chemotherapy
    I. Title
    616.9'94061
Library of Congress Control Number: 2007936871

ISBN: 978-1-84628-989-7   e-ISBN: 978-1-84628-991-0

Printed on acid-free paper

9 8 7 6 5 4 3 2 1

Springer Science+Business Media
springer.com

Preface

This book is intended as a basic overview of the drug treatment of cancer for junior doctors and specialist nurses who come into contact with people having chemotherapy as part of their day-to-day work. The aim is to provide a context to those treatments, explaining what the drugs are, how they work, some of their more likely side effects, how they are used in the treatment of the commoner cancers and what therapeutic results might be expected.

The first use of the word chemotherapy is credited to Paul Ehrlich (1854–1915), who used it to describe the arsenical compounds he developed to treat syphilis. Nowadays when people talk about 'chemotherapy', as part of cancer treatment, they are usually referring to the use of cytotoxic drugs. Cytotoxics have dominated systemic cancer therapy for the last 50 years, and their use has resulted in enormous improvements in outcome. But they are only one component of the drug treatment of malignancy. Hormonal therapies are another major contributor to increased cure rates and survival times, and the last decade has seen an explosion of entirely new types of drugs for cancer treatment. The latter are mainly drugs specifically targeted against cancer cells (whereas cytotoxics affect both normal and malignant cells). These newer compounds have sometimes been popularly termed 'magic bullets', which again takes us back to Ehrlich, as this was another phrase he used to describe his treatments.

The aim of this text is to cover all these different elements of systemic therapy, giving an explanation of their various modes of action, their side effects and their place in the everyday treatment of common cancers, with the hope of offering a simple overview of an increasingly complex, diverse, and incredibly exciting area of modern-day medicine.

While some cytotoxic and hormonal agents have been in common use for more than 50 years, many of the treatments described in this book have only appeared in the last 5 years, and others remain prospects for the future. The recent rapid expansion of therapeutic options for systemic cancer treatment, with drugs having a range of new lines of attack on the process of cancer growth, has meant that there is no universally agreed system for classifying these therapies. Because some of the newer agents only affect cancer cells, and cause relatively little damage to normal tissue (in contrast to the established cytotoxic drugs), they have been called 'targeted' therapies. Another phrase that is used is 'biological therapies' or 'biological response modifiers'; some authorities restrict this to describing the cytokines, whilst others use it to embrace a far wider range of compounds, including all the monoclonal antibodies. As a result the current terminology can be confusing and is still evolving. I have adopted the approach of trying to show how all these different options we now have for attacking cancer relate to the basic process of tumour growth and development.

Details of specific drug doses and treatment schedules are deliberately not given. This is partly because there is often considerable variation from hospital to hospital on the precise dosage and timing of treatment, even with 'standard' therapies. But also the prescription of most of the drugs described in this book is restricted to experienced specialist clinicians and would not normally be the responsibility of more junior doctors. So whilst it is important to be aware of what the drugs are and why they are being used, it is not anticipated that the readers of this book would be involved in either the choice treatment or its prescription.

Throughout the text I have used the approved (non-proprietary) names of the drugs. The UK proprietary (trade) names are given in Appendix 1.

A current complication of cancer chemotherapy in the UK is the drug approval process. Once a new agent has gained its commercial product licence it may be prescribed. However, until the drug has been approved by the National Institute for Health and Clinical Excellence (NICE), in England and Wales, and the Scottish Medicines Consortium, in Scotland it will not be available on the National Health Service (NHS). This system, designed to ensure cost effectiveness of therapeutic innovations, is not without its critics – not least because the two authorities sometimes reach different decisions! However, it does mean that at the time of writing some of the newer drugs mentioned in the text either are still awaiting approval or, for the present at least, have failed to gain approval. Because this is a constantly changing situation and because most of the readers of this book would not be directly involved in selecting treatments, I have specifically avoided commenting on the availability, or otherwise, of drugs on the NHS.

Throughout the text I have given suggestions for further reading, citing articles which cover individual topics in more depth. In addition there are three textbooks which give more detailed accounts of almost all the subjects I have covered, and which provide excellent references. They are *Cancer Chemotherapy and Biotherapy*, 4th edition, Chabner BA, Longo DL, eds, Lippincott, Williams and Wilkins, 2006; *Cancer: Principles and Practice of Oncology*, 7th edition, DeVita DT, Hellman S, Rosenberg SA, eds, Lippincott Williams & Wilkins, 2005; *The Oxford Textbook of Oncology*, 2nd edition, Souhami RL, Tannock I, Hohenberger P, Horiot J-C, eds, Oxford University Press, 2002.

Terry Priestman
May 2007

Contents

Part I
The Theoretical Basis of Cancer Chemotherapy

HISTORICAL INTRODUCTION

The first drugs to treat cancer effectively were the hormonal and cytotoxic agents which appeared in the early 1940s.

In 1896 the Glasgow surgeon, George Beatson, reported the remission of an advanced breast cancer in a young woman, following removal of her ovaries. In a parallel discovery, just over 40 years later, Charles Huggins, working in Chicago, showed that prostate cancer would regress following castration. Shortly before this, in 1938, Charles Dodds, in London, had produced a synthetic form of the female hormone oestrogen: stilboestrol. In 1941 Huggins showed that, stilboestrol could cause prostate cancer to regress, and in 1944 Alexander Haddow reported the successful use of the drug to treat women with metastatic breast cancer.

At the same time, other pioneers were building on the First World War observation that the poison gas, sulphur mustard, caused shrinkage of lymphoid tissue, and a fall in the white blood cell count, as well as many other effects. In 1942 Goodman and Gilman, working at Yale, used nitrogen mustard, a derivative of sulphur mustard, to treat a man with advanced lymphoma: his cancer briefly regressed.

Stilboestrol and nitrogen mustard opened the flood gates, and over the last 60 years more than a 100 hormonal and cytotoxic agents have been developed for cancer treatment.

These early breakthroughs were based on empirical observations, why the treatments worked was a mystery. Relatively quickly, it was realized that nitrogen mustard, and the numerous other cytotoxic agents that followed in its wake, acted by directly interfering with the process of cell division – inhibiting mitosis in one way or another. But it was not until the 1958 that Elwood

Jensen discovered oestrogen receptors (ER), providing a basis for understanding the hormonal sensitivity of some cancers.

We now know that about two out of three breast cancers are made up of cells carrying ER (ER+ cancers). Those ER bind circulating oestrogen, and in so doing are stimulated to promote cell division: the cancer is hormone dependent for its growth. In the same way, it has been discovered that most prostate cancers carry receptors for the male hormone, androgen, and this drives their growth.

The receptor story gives us an insight into more recent developments in the drug treatment of cancer. In 1977 the epidermal growth factor receptor (EGFR) was identified, the first of a number of tyrosine kinase receptors which have been found in many different types of cancer. This has led to the development of at least three lines of therapeutic attack. The first of these has focused on reducing the levels of circulating growth factors which stimulate these receptors. The second approach has been to explore ways of blocking or inhibiting receptors, so they cannot be stimulated. The third approach has looked at the next stage in the pathway of cell growth: when a receptor is stimulated it then sends a message to the cell nucleus, telling it to make the cell divide. This is known as signal transduction. Much research in recent years has been focused on identifying the chemical messengers that link the receptor to the nucleus, carrying the signals for cell division, and now the first drugs are appearing that can disrupt these chemicals, and break the chain of communication between the receptor and the nucleus.

This brief history identifies the key milestones in the development of cancer chemotherapy. It also indicates how the discovery of new systemic treatments for cancer has been paralleled by an increasing understanding of tumour biology. The latter now gives us a clear picture of the natural history of cancers, from their origin, at a molecular level, in genetic mutations, to the impact those changes have on the mechanisms controlling cell growth, and a knowledge of subsequent tumour kinetics, which leads to the appearance of clinically obvious, potentially lethal, malignancies. To fill in more detail about the types of anti-cancer drugs that are used now, and might be used in the future, and to explain how they work the approach we will adopt is to look at the natural history of cancer, and relate the different types of systemic therapy to the various stages of cancer development (Fig. 1.1).

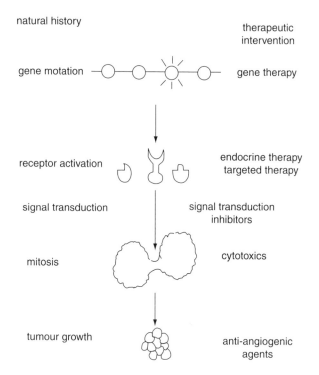

FIGURE 1.1. The natural history of cancer and the place of different chemotherapeutic interventions.

Suggestions for further reading

Chabner BA, Roberts TG. Chemotherapy and the war on cancer. Nature Rev Cancer, 2005; 5: 65–72.

Hirsch J. An anniversary for cancer chemotherapy. JAMA 2006; 296: 1518–1520.

Thomas A. Joe Burchenal and the birth of combination chemotherapy. Br J Haematol, 2006; 133: 493–503.

IN THE BEGINNING: GENES

Cancers begin as the result of an abnormality in the genes of one or more cells in the body. That abnormality may either be inherited, the faulty gene being passed from one generation to the next, or acquired, a normal gene being damaged or mutating for some reason.

Two types of genes have been identified which have a role in cancer formation: oncogenes and tumour suppressor genes. When an oncogene mutates it switches on the process of uncontrolled cell division which leads to a cancer. Tumour suppressor genes, as their name implies, normally regulate the process of cell replication, keeping it under control, when they mutate that control is lost, the brakes are off, and once again uncontrolled cell division occurs.

The first gene to be shown to be directly related to cancer development was the *RB-1*, retinoblastoma, gene, abnormalities of which lead to the childhood cancer of the same name, which affects the retina. This is a rare tumour, but among the more common cancers we now know about 1 in 20 breast cancers result from mutations in either the *BRCA1* or the *BRCA2* gene, and about 1 in 25 bowel cancers result from changes in the *FPC* (familial polyposis coli) gene, or the *HNPC* (hereditary non-polyposis coli) gene. As it happens, all these are tumour suppressor genes. At the present time an ever increasing number of genes are being discovered, mutations of which may lead to cancer.

The identification of these genetic abnormalities opens the way for a whole new approach to cancer treatment: gene therapy. There are a number of ways in which this could be used (Table 1.1) but at the moment these are very much at the research stage, either in the laboratory or in the most preliminary of clinical trials. It will be some years until we know whether targeting genes will produce results, but already some enthusiasts

TABLE 1.1. Some ways in which anti-cancer gene therapy might be used

Replacing faulty genes: inserting new normal genes into the cells to replace the abnormal cancerous genes.

Boosting immunity: altering the cancer genes to make their cells more vulnerable to the body's immune system.

Increasing sensitivity to treatment: altering the cancer genes to make their cells either more vulnerable to other treatments, or to stop them developing resistance to those treatments.

Reducing the sensitivity of normal cells to treatment: selectively targeting normal genes to make their cells more resistant to the effects of treatment, so that higher doses of drugs or radiation may be given.

Suicide genes: introducing genes into cancer cells which are designed to destroy the abnormal oncogenes or tumour suppressor genes.

Anti-angiogenesis genes: introducing genes into cancer cells that will stop them from developing the new blood vessels essential for the support of tumour growth.

are claiming that within a generation gene therapy will have virtually eliminated cancer.

Suggestion for further reading

Lattime EC, Gerson S. Introduction: gene therapy of cancer. Semin Oncol, 2005; 32: 535–537. (This whole issue of the journal is devoted to gene therapy of cancer and gives a comprehensive overview of the subject.)

GROWTH FACTORS AND RECEPTORS

We all begin our lives as a single fertilized cell. That cell then divides to form two cells, those two cells divide to make four, and this process of cell division continues throughout pregnancy, and on through infancy, childhood and adolescence, to produce the countless billions of cells that make up our adult selves. The process of cell growth continues in adulthood, because cells are constantly wearing out and dying off and need to be replaced. Throughout our lives, this process of cell division is very precisely controlled so that we make exactly the right number of new cells that our bodies need – no more, no less. A cancer develops when the cells in a particular organ escape from these controls and begin to reproduce and grow in a haphazard way, producing more cells than they should.

Key components of the control process for cell division are growth factors and receptors. Growth factors are chemicals which circulate in the blood stream and bind to specific receptor sites on the cell surface or in the cellular cytoplasm. The resulting interaction between the growth factor and the receptor then triggers the next step in stimulating cell division.

Faulty genes can affect the growth factor–receptor system in a number of ways. For example, they can cause an overproduction, or over-expression, of growth factor receptors. This effectively makes the cell far more sensitive to natural growth factors, which stimulate them to multiply excessively. Alternatively they may lead receptors to be active even when they are not being stimulated by growth factors.

At the present time the two families of receptors that are of major importance in oncology are steroid receptors and the tyrosine kinase receptors.

STEROID RECEPTORS AND ENDOCRINE THERAPY

The two main steroid receptors related to cancer growth are oestrogen and androgen receptors. About two out of three breast cancers are made up of cells carrying an abnormally high level of oestrogen receptors, they are ER+, similarly more than 9 out of 10 prostate cancers have an over expression of androgen receptors. These receptor-positive cancers rely on circulating hormone to stimulate their growth. Oestrogen or androgen interact with the receptors to produce chemical signals which trigger the process of mitosis (Fig. 1.2).

Oestrogen and androgen could be thought of as the first cancer growth factors to be recognized, although they are not normally classified in that way.

Therapeutically this hormonally driven cancer growth can be inhibited in two ways: either by reducing the level of circulating hormone or by blocking the receptor so that the hormonal growth factor cannot reach it. In pre-menopausal women, circulating oestrogen levels may be reduced either by inhibition of sex hormone production by the pituitary gland (using gonaderilin analogues) or by ablation of the ovaries, by surgery or radiotherapy. The gonaderilin analogues (also known

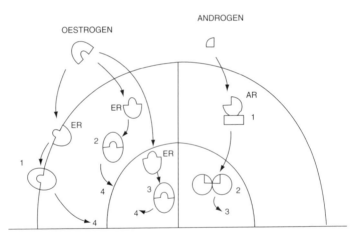

FIGURE 1.2. Oestrogen and androgen receptor signalling pathways
Circulating oestrogen binds to oestrogen receptors (ER) in the cell membrane, in the cytoplasm or in the nucleus to form membrane (1), mitochondrial (2) or nuclear (3) oestrogen–receptor complexes, which then trigger the release of signalling proteins (4) to stimulate DNA synthesis and cell division. Androgen receptors (AR) are in the cytoplasm, bound to a protein which inactivates them (1). Androgen releases the receptor from the protein and it moves to the cell nucleus where receptors form pairs (dimerize) (2) and bind to androgen-response elements which trigger the release of signalling proteins to stimulate DNA synthesis and cell division (3).

as LHRH, luteinizing hormone-releasing hormone, analogues) initially stimulate pituitary receptors, leading to a transient increase in luteinizing hormone, and hence sex hormone, levels, before down-regulating the receptors, rendering them insensitive. Although ovarian production of oestrogen ceases with the menopause, the hormone is still produced elsewhere in the body, especially in the fatty tissues, where androgen secreted by the adrenal gland is converted into oestrogen (Fig. 1.3). This synthesis involves the aromatase enzymes, and their inhibition leads to a fall in oestrogen levels. So the aromatase inhibitors are drugs which reduce oestrogen levels in older women. By contrast, tamoxifen acts at all ages by blocking the oestrogen receptor itself. This statement is a slight oversimplification of tamoxifen's action, although it does competitively block ER on cancer cells, it actually has a stimulatory effect on other ER, for example those in the endometrium lining the womb. This more complex relationship with ER is reflected in an alternative description of tamoxifen as a selective oestrogen receptor modulator (SERM). A new drug, fulvestrant, also works by attacking ER, down-regulating, and effectively inactivating the receptor.

Another group of hormones active in breast cancer are the progestogens, synthetic forms of the female hormone progesterone. Although some breast cancer cells do carry specific progestogen receptors (PgR+ cancers), the interaction of the drugs with these is probably of secondary importance in their anti-tumour effect as they also have a number of other properties including reducing ovarian and adrenal androgen production, reducing the expression of ER, and, possibly, a direct cytotoxic action on breast cancer cells.

In prostate cancer, gonaderilin analogues or surgical castration maybe used to reduce circulating androgen levels, whilst anti-androgenic agents mimic the action of tamoxifen in competing for receptors on the cancer cell. These latter drugs are classified as either steroidal (cyproterone acetate) or non-steroidal (flutamide, bicalutamide). Because of its steroidal properties, cyproterone also causes some pituitary inhibition of hormone production as well as the competitive inhibition of androgen receptors. A consequence of these slightly differing modes of action is that the non-steroidal anti-androgens do not lower circulating androgen levels whilst cyproterone does, and this affects the side-effect profile of the drugs (see P. 73). In the early days of systemic therapy for prostate cancer, stilboestrol was the drug of choice. This acts in a number of ways, including reduction of LHRH secretion, inactivation

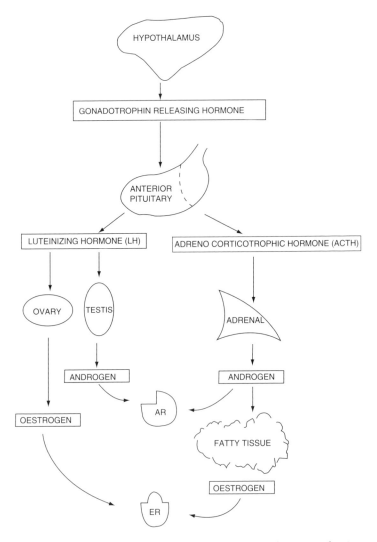

FIGURE 1.3. Hormonal pathways for oestrogen and androgen production
Before the menopause luteinizing hormone (LH) stimulates production of
androgen in the ovary which is converted to oestrogen by the aromatase
enzyme pathway. After the menopause oestrogen production continues, at
a much reduced level, by conversion of androgen secreted by the adrenals
carried out by aromatase enzymes mainly in the fatty tissues.

TABLE 1.2. Hormonal agents

Mode of action	Breast cancer	Prostate cancer
Gonaderilin analogues	goserelin	goserelin leuprorelin
Competitive receptor inhibitors	tamoxifen toremifene	bicalutamide cyproterone flutamide
Receptor downregulation	fulvestrant	
Aromatase inhibition	anastrazole exemestane letrozole	
Multiple modes of action	progestogens: megestrol acetate medroxyprogesterone acetate	diethyl- stilboestrol

of circulating androgen and direct suppression of androgen production by the testes; it has also been suggested that it may be directly cytotoxic to tumour cells in the prostate. Although the drug fell out of favour for many years because of a high level of thromboembolic complications, it has now regained a place as an effective third- or fourth- line treatment in metastatic prostate cancer.

Another family of hormone receptors is the glucocorticoid receptors. These are found in the cytoplasm of lymphocytes and are the target of the corticosteroids prednisone, prednisolone and dexamethasone. When the corticosteroid binds to the receptors the steroid–receptor complex moves to the cell nucleus and activates programmed cell death (apoptosis). In this way, giving steroids reduces the number of lymphocytes, and this forms the basis for their use in a number of haematological cancers.

Suggestions for further reading

Debes JD, Tindall DJ. Mechanisms of androgen-refractory prostate cancer. New Engl J Med, 2004; 351: 1488–1490.

Chmelar R, Buchanan G, Need EF et al. Androgen receptor coregulators and their involvement in the development and progression of prostate cancer. Int J Cancer, 2007; 120: 719–733.

Sharifi N, Gulley JL, Dahut WL. Androgen deprivation therapy for prostate cancer. JAMA, 2005; 294: 238–244.

Yager JD, Davidson NE. Estrogen carcinogenesis in breast cancer. New Engl J Med, 2006; 354: 270–282.

TYROSINE KINASE GENES

The human genome contains more than 100 tyrosine kinase (TK) genes. These genes produce tyrosine kinases which are a family of enzymes involved in the regulation of cell division (mitosis), programmed cell death (apoptosis) and a number of other cellular functions. There are a number of different families of *TK* genes, and three of these in particular play a crucial part in the growth of certain cancers, these are the epidermal growth factor receptors (EGFR), vascular endothelial growth factor receptors (VEGFR) and non-receptor tyrosine kinases. The EGF and VEGF receptors have similar structure, as shown in Fig. 1.4.

EGFR

EGFRs are a family of receptors made up of EGFR, HER2, HER3 and HER4. EGFRs are found in normal epithelial cells, and are stimulated by a number of different growth factors, the two most important of which are epidermal growth factor (EGF) and transforming growth factor α (TGF-α). Incidentally the compounds which bind to, and stimulate, these receptors are often referred to as ligands.

EGFRs are made up of three parts or domains: an extracellular domain, which binds the circulating growth factors, a transmembrane domain, which crosses the cell membrane and an intracellular (tyrosine kinase) domain. Stimulation causes the

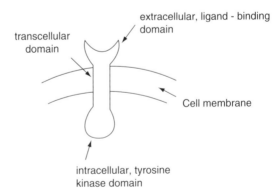

FIGURE 1.4. The basic structure of a tyrosine kinase (TK) receptor The extracellular domain is the target for monoclonal antibodies like cetuximab, bevacizumab or trastuzumab. The intracellular domain is the target for small molecule TK inhibitors like erlotinib, gefitinib and lapatinib.

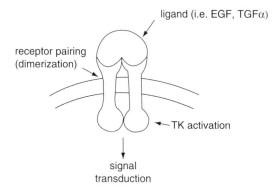

FIGURE 1.5. Activation of EGFR family receptors
Dimerization may be between two of the same receptors, that is EGFR and EGFR (homodimerization), or two different receptors, that is EGFR and HER2 (heterodimerization). HER2 has no known ligands and is activated by heterodimerization, although if HER2 is heavily over-expressed it can form homodimers which can activate the TK signalling pathway without ligand binding (autoactivation). The intracellular domain of HER3 has no TK component, but HER3 can activate signal transduction by forming heterodimers with other EGFRs.

receptors to form into pairs (this is called dimerization). Dimerization leads to a change in the structure of the receptors which then triggers the intracellular domain to activate a biochemical pathway in which the tyrosine kinase enzymes are the key component (Fig. 1.5).

Both EGFR1 and EGFR2 have been linked to a number of cancers (Table 1.3). Genetic mutations can affect these receptors in a number of ways, the most important of which is over expression, producing an excess of the receptors in the cell, which makes that cell abnormally sensitive to circulating growth factors.

Looking for drugs that will inhibit the EGFR system is one of the most active areas of research in oncology at present. So far two types of agent have been developed: monoclonal antibodies, which bind to and block the extracellular receptor domain, and small-molecule EGFR tyrosine kinase inhibitors (TKIs), which suppress the activation of the intracellular domain (Table 1.4).

VEGFR and Related Receptors
Once a cancer begins to grow then in order to survive it needs to develop its own blood supply. This involves creating new blood vessels, a process known as angiogenesis. The cells which form the

TABLE 1.3. The epidermal growth factor receptor family

Receptor	Alternative names	Over-expressed in these cancers
EGFR	HER1* erbB1[†] ErbB1	Head and neck (90%) Kidney, clear cell (70%) Lung, non-small cell (60%) Breast, ovary, colorectal (50%) Pancreas, bladder, prostate (40%)
HER2	erbB2 ErbB2 HER2/neu c-erbB-2	Breast (20%) Endometrial (15%) Ovary Cervical (15%)
HER3	erbB3 ErbB3	Breast, colon, stomach, prostate, soft tissue sarcoma
HER4	erbB4 ErbB4	Breast, prostate, medulloblastoma

* HER: an abbreviation of human epidermal growth factor.
[†] erbB: this has its origin in the fact that EGFR was discovered through work on oncogenes present in the avian erythroblastosis gene (v-erbB).

capillaries are the endothelial cells. More than a dozen different chemicals have been identified that can be formed by cancers to stimulate angiogenesis. Three of the most important of these are vascular endothelial growth factor (VEGF), basic fibroblast growth factor (βFGF) and platelet-derived growth factor (PDGF). VEGF binds to two different receptors, VEGF

TABLE 1.4. EGFR family inhibitors

Drug	Type	Receptor/domain targeted	Formulation
Cetuximab	moab*	EGFR/extracellular	iv
Trastuzumab	moab	HER2/extracellular	iv
Pertuzumab	moab	HER2/extracellular	iv
Gefitinib	TK1[†]	EGFR/intracellular	oral
Erlotinib	TK1	EGFR/intracellular	oral
Lapatinib	TK1	EGFR & HER2/intracellular	oral
Canertinib	TK1	EGFR & HER2/intracellular	oral

* Monoclonal antibody.
[†] Small molecule tyrosine kinase inhibitor.

receptor type 1 and 2 (VEGFR-1, and VEGFR-2), and βFGF and PDGF both have their own receptors.

VEGF, βFGF and PDGF activation of their receptors stimulates tyrosine kinase activity which, among other things, releases enzymes called matrix metalloproteinases (MMPs) which breakdown the extracellular matrix: the supportive material that holds the cells together. This allows the endothelial cells to spread and multiply, thereby forming new blood vessels.

Looking for agents that will suppress tumour angiogenesis is another current major research area, and once again monoclonal antibodies neutralizing endothelial growth factors, or blocking their receptors, have been developed as well as small-molecule tyrosine kinase inhibitors. As well as these agents that target the endothelial growth factor–receptor system other compounds are available, or in development which attack other aspects of the tumour vascularity. Collectively these drugs are known as anti-angiogenic agents, and they are summarized in Fig. 1.6. Imatinib, sorafenib and sunitinib are of particular note as they are multi-targeted drugs, inhibiting a number of different components of the tyrosine kinase system (Table 1.5). One particularly interesting member of this group is thalidomide, which achieved notoriety in the 1960s when its use in the treatment

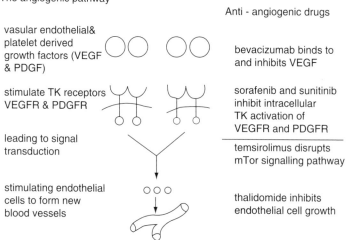

The angiogenic pathway

Anti - angiogenic drugs

vasular endothelial& platelet derived growth factors (VEGF & PDGF)

bevacizumab binds to and inhibits VEGF

stimulate TK receptors VEGFR & PDGFR

sorafenib and sunitinib inhibit intracellular TK activation of VEGFR and PDGFR

leading to signal transduction

temsirolimus disrupts mTor signalling pathway

stimulating endothelial cells to form new blood vessels

thalidomide inhibits endothelial cell growth

FIGURE 1.6. The inhibition of tumour angiogenesis.
Note: Although not its main mode of action, imatinib is also an inhibitor of PDGFR.

TABLE 1.5. Targeted therapies: multi-targeted drugs

Drug	Targets	Therapeutic indications
Imatinib	BCR-ABL KIT** PDGFR	Chronic myeloid leukaemia Gastrointestinal stromal tumours (GIST)
Sorafenib	VEGFR PDGFR KIT MAPK/Ras	Renal cell cancer Prostate cancer* Head and neck cancer* Melanoma*
Sunitinib	VEGFR PDGFR KIT RET[†]	Renal cell cancer GIST* Breast cancer* Neuroendocrine tumours*

* Currently under investigation, value to be established.
** A tyrosine kinase over expressed in some leukaemias and GIST
[†] A receptor linked to some neuroendocrine tumours.

of morning sickness during pregnancy resulted in the birth defect phocomelia (failure of development of the long bones). This toxicity was in part due to its anti-angiogenic activity in the developing embryo, which is now being capatilized on in the treatment of multiple myeloma and being explored in other cancers. Thalidomide inhibits the transcription of angiogenic genes and thus prevents the formation of chemicals stimulating the process of new blood vessel formation. Apart from its teratogenic potential, thalidomide does have other side effects, including peripheral neuropathy, drowsiness and constipation. Recently a related drug, lenalidomide, has been developed which appears to have similar anti-angiogenic properties to thalidomide, but with fewer side effects.

Non-receptor Tyrosine Kinases
Unlike the EGF and VEGF receptors these tyrosine kinases exist in the cytoplasm, not on the surface of the cell, and have no receptor sites. Therefore they are not activated by the binding of a growth factor, or ligand, but as a result of some cellular abnormality which leads to autostimulation, producing growth-signalling proteins in the absence of any external stimulus. This mechanism has been most clearly demonstrated in a number of haematological cancers, where it occurs as a result of chromosomal translocations. The best studied of these is in chronic myeloid leukaemia, where 95% of patients have a translocation

between chromosomes 9 and 22, producing what is known as the Philadelphia chromosome. This translocation produces a fusion gene, *brc-abl*, which in turn stimulates a specific non-receptor tyrosine kinase pathway, BCR-ABL, which causes the leukaemic change. This process can be disrupted by the drug imatinib, which is an inhibitor of ABL and a number of ABL-related gene products.

Suggestions for further reading

Eskens F. Angiogenesis inhibitors in clinical development; where are we now and where are we going? Br J Cancer, 2004; 90: 1–7.

Faivre S, Djellloul S, Raymond E. New paradigms in anticancer therapy: targeting multiple signalling pathways with kinase inhibitors. Semin Oncol, 2006; 33: 407–420.

Gross ME, Shazer RL, Agus DB. Targeting the HER-kinase axis in cancer. Semin Oncol, 2004; 31 (suppl 3): 9–20.

Krause DS, Van Etten RA. Tyrosine kinases as targets for cancer therapy. N Engl J Med, 2005; 353: 172–187.

Marshall J. Clinical implications of the mechanism of epidermal growth factor receptor inhibitors. Cancer, 2006; 107: 1207–1218.

Mendelsohn J, Baselga J. Epidermal growth factor receptor targeting in cancer. Semin Oncol, 2006; 33: 369–385.

CYTOKINES

Another group of compounds that could be considered as growth factors are the cytokines. Cytokines are an extensive family of naturally occurring proteins which play a part in regulating various aspects of the immune system, as well as a number of other physiological functions. Two cytokines have emerged as agents for anti-cancer therapy: interferon and interleukin. There is still controversy over the exact way in which these compounds affect cancer cells: some experts argue for a direct effect, whilst others suggest that they work by stimulating the immune system to attack the cancer. These uncertainties are reflected in the confusing terminology for these agents which have been referred to variously as biological response modifiers, biological therapies, immunomodulators or, simply, immunotherapy.

CD PROTEIN–TARGETED MONOCLONAL ANTIBODIES

Another group of biological therapies are monoclonal antibodies designed to target proteins on normal and malignant B lymphocytes. The two compounds currently licensed in the UK are rituximab and alemtuzumab, they target the CD20 and CD52 proteins respectively. These proteins are found on the surface of normal and malignant cells, but are not present on normal stem cells, so that normal cells are readily replaced, with a minimum of toxicity. The monoclonal antibodies bind to the proteins, and this binding then acts as a signal to normal immune mechanisms to destroy the cells.

SIGNAL TRANSDUCTION

Once a receptor has been stimulated it stimulates cell growth by sending a message to the cell nucleus which will lead to either mitosis or inhibition of apoptosis. For steroid receptors there are a number of pathways but the classical interaction is a direct one, with hormones binding to receptors located in the cell nucleus. The EGFR and VEGFR families of receptors, located on the cell membrane, have to produce chemical messengers to travel to the nucleus to relay their stimulus. This process is called signal transduction. Once again multiple tyrosine kinase pathways play a key part in this process, and as these become identified so drugs can be developed to target them. Three signalling cascades have been identified as particularly important in cancer development, they are

1. mitogen-activated protein kinase (MAPK/Ras)
2. phosphatidyl inositol-3-kinase (PI3K/AKT)
3. protein kinase C (PKC).

Many drugs are under development as potential inhibitors of these pathways. Those which have reached advanced stages in clinical trials are temsirolimus and sorafenib. Temsirolimus inhibits the protein mTOR, which is a key component in the PI3K/AKT pathway. Sorafenib inhibits Raf kinase, which is a key enzyme in the MAPK/ras signal transduction cascade. Like imatinib and sunitinib, sorafenib is a multi-targeted drug, also inhibiting VEGF, PDGF and KIT receptors. Another group of drugs which are under development are the farnesyl transferase inhibitors. Farnesyl transferase is another key enzyme in the MAPK/Ras pathway.

Suggestion for further reading
Schreck R, Rapp VR. Raf kinases: oncogenesis and drug discovery. Int J Cancer, 2006; 119: 2261–2271.

PROTEASOME INHIBITION

Proteasomes are enzyme complexes which are present in all cells. They degrade proteins that control a number of cellular activities, including the regulation of cell division. Inhibition of the proteasome interferes with the chemical signals which stimulate cell growth and replication. Cancer cells appear to be more sensitive to disturbance of proteasome function than normal cells. The first proteasome inhibitor to have been approved is bortezomib, which has been shown to be of value in the treatment of multiple myeloma. Other proteasome inhibitors are in development and the proteasome is likely to be an increasingly important target for new cancer drugs.

Suggestion for further reading

Leonard JP, Furman RR, Coleman M. Proteasome inhibition with borte-
    zomib: a new therapeutic strategy for non-Hodgkin's lymphoma. Int J
    Cancer, 2006; 119: 971–979.
Mitchell BS. The proteasome – an emerging therapeutic target in cancer.
    New Engl J Med, 2003; 348: 2597–2598.

MITOSIS: CYTOTOXIC DRUGS

We now reach the stage in the carcinogenic pathway where the cell is stimulated to multiply in an uncontrolled fashion. The mechanism for that multiplication is the fundamental process of mitosis, with the duplication of the nuclear genetic material on the chromosomes and the subsequent formation of two new daughter cells from the original one. This is the point at which the classical cytotoxic chemotherapy drugs, the compounds which have evolved from the discovery of nitrogen mustard, take effect.

Cytotoxic drugs all act by disrupting the process of mitosis. They do this in a variety of ways, and their mode of action forms a basis for their classification (Table 1.6).

Because cytotoxic drugs are still the major component of systemic anti-cancer therapy, it is appropriate to describe here the mode of action of the main groups of drugs in a little more detail.

Alkylating Agents

Nitrogen mustard, the first cytotoxic drug to be identified in the 1940s (see p. 1) is an alkylating agent. Within 20 years of its first application more than 3,000 other alkylating agents had been isolated for evaluation in cancer treatment. Of these 3,000, only a handful are in general use today.

An alkyl group is the chemical structure that results when an aliphatic or aromatic hydrocarbon loses one of its hydrogen atoms. The simplest of all alkyl groups has the formula CH_2. An alkylating agent is a compound that contains an alkyl group and is able to use that group to combine with other compounds

TABLE 1.6. A classification of cytotoxic drugs in common use

Alkylating agents

Busulfan	Melphalan
Carmustine	Mitomycin*
Chlorambucil	Nitrogen mustard
Cyclophosphamide	Procarbazine
Dacarbazine	Temozolamide
Ifosfamide	Thiotepa
Lomustine	Treosulfan

Platinum analogues

Carboplatin	Oxaliplatin
Cisplatin	

Antimetabolites

Captecitabine	Mercaptopurine
Cladribine	Methotrexate
Cytaribine	Pemetrexed
Fludarabine	Pentostatin
Fluorouracil	Raltitrexed '
Gemcitabine	Tegafur with uracil
Hydroxyurea	Thioguanine

Topoisomerase I inhibitors

Irinotecan	Topotecan

Topoisomerase II inhibitors

Amsacrine	Etoposide
Daunorubicin*	Idarubicin*
Doxorubicin*	Mitoxantrone*
Epirubicin	

Cytotoxic antibiotics

Bleomycin	Dactinomycin

Anti-microtubule drugs

Docetaxel	Vincristine
Paclitaxel	Vindesine
Vinblastine	Vinorelbine

* May also be classified as cytotoxic antibitotics.

by covalent bonds. At its simplest the general formula for an alkylating reaction or alkylation is

$$R - CH_2 - X + Y = R - CH_2 - Y + X$$

The principal action of cytotoxic alkylating agents is to attack the nitrogen atom at the N-7 position on the purine base guanine, in DNA and RNA. Most of the drugs possess not one but two alkyl groups, and are termed bifunctional alkylating agents. The molecular distance between the two alkyl groups is such that they can each bind to a guanine base on the strands on the DNA chain where a turn in the helix brings them close together. In this way the alkylating agents form bridges, or cross-linkages, between the DNA strands which prevent them from separating at the time of DNA replication prior to cell division. In addition at those points in the DNA chain where separation does occur the alkylating agents will attach to any free guanine bases and prevent them from acting as templates for the formation of new DNA (this is a major mode of action for monofunctional alkylating agents, containing only one alkyl group, which are not able to form cross-linkages). In this way DNA replication and hence subsequent cell division are inhibited.

The alkylating agents can be grouped into a number of classes based on their chemical properties, and these are shown in Table 1.7.

Platinum Analogues

Cisplatin was developed following the observation, in 1965, that passing an electric current between platinum electrodes in nutrient broth inhibited the growth of bacteria. As a result cisplatin was developed, which is a complex of chlorine and ammonia ions with platinum. Following intracellular activation

TABLE 1.7. Classification of commonly used cytotoxic alkylating agents

Nitrogen mustards	
Chlorambucil	Melphalan
Cyclophosphamide	Nitrogen mustard
Ifosfamide	
Nitrosoureas	
Carmustine	Lomustine
Alkylalkanesulfonates	
Busulfan	Treosulfan
Aziridines	
Mitomycin *	Thiotepa
Tetrazines	
Dacarbazine **	Temozolomide [†]
Procarbazine**	

* Also classed as a cytotixic antibitoitc.
[†] Monofunctional akylating agents.

cisplatin forms cross linkages with DNA, mainly by attacking the N-7 moiety of the guanine, thus acting like a bifunctional alkylating agent. Indeed, in some classifications, the platinum compounds are classed as alkylating agents.

Following the discovery of cisplatin, analogues have been produced, of which the two in common use are carboplatin and oxaliplatin, and further similar drugs are currently under development.

Ant-metabolites

The antimetabolites were the second family of cytotoxics to be discovered and were first used in the Unites States in the late 1940s. They work as follows: before a cell can divide it must build up large reserves of nucleic acid and protein. For this synthesis to take place various metabolites must be present to form the subunits from which the larger molecules will be built and enzymes must be available to achieve the synthesis. The antimetabolites may either be chemical analogues of the essential subunits, which then get incorporated into DNA in their place, making faulty DNA which prevents successful cell division, or they may be inhibitors of vital enzymes.

To understand the way the individual cytotoxic antimetabolites work, it might be helpful to recap on two bits of basic cell biology: the composition of DNA and the importance of folic acid. DNA is made up of thousands of subunits called nucleotides, and each nucleotide has three components – a phosphate group; a five carbon (pentose) sugar, deoxyribose; and a nitrogen containing base (Fig. 1.7). The base may be one of two purines (adenine or guanine) or pyrimidines (cytosine or thymine) (Fig. 1.8). Folic acid is a vitamin essential for normal cell growth. After a number of enzymatic conversions in the body it appears in its biologically active form as folinic acid. Folinic acid is an essential co-enzyme in the synthesis of purines and pyrimidines. The second stage in the conversion of folic acid to folinic acid is the transformation of

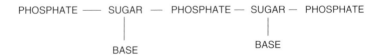

PHOSPHATE —— SUGAR — PHOSPHATE — SUGAR — PHOSPHATE

BASE   BASE

FIGURE 1.7. The structure of the DNA chain.
The sugar is deoxyribose, and the bases are the pyrimidines, cytosine and thymine, and the purines, guanine and adenine.

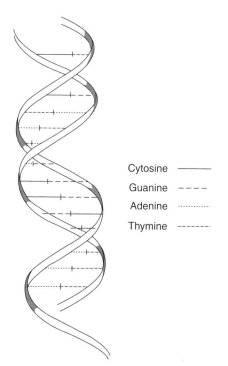

Cytosine ——————
Guanine – – – –
Adenine ·············
Thymine ---------

FIGURE 1.8. The DNA complex.
Two DNA chains are linked in a spiral structure by hydrogen bonds between base pairs. These bonds are highly specific: adenine can only unite with thymine and guanine can only unite with cytosine.

dihydrofolate to tetrahydrofolate. This transformation is carried out by the enzyme dihydrofolate reductase.

The commonly used antimetabolites can be placed into three groups: those which inhibit the conversion of folic acid to folinic acid (and hence inhibit purine and pyrimidine synthesis), those which interfere with purine synthesis, and those which interfere with pyrimidine synthesis. The groups are as follows:

- Drugs inhibiting folinic acid production: methotrexate, pemetrexed, and raltitrexed.
- Drugs interfering with purine synthesis: mercaptopurine, thioguanine, fludarabine, cladribine, hydroxyurea and pentostatin.
- Drugs interfering with pyrimidine synthesis: fluorouracil, capecitabine, gemcitabine, cytaribine, and tegafur with uracil.

Leucovorin (calcium folinate, folinic acid) is an interesting compound in relation to the antimetabolites, in that it acts to both increase the efficacy of fluororacil and reduce the toxicity of methotrexate. The active metabolites of fluorouracil work by inhibiting the enzyme thimdylate synthase, but bind only relatively weakly with this enzyme. Leucovorin strengthens this binding, and so prolongs the duration of fluorouracil's anti-cancer activity. The combination of fluorouracil and leucovorin has been used mainly in colorectal cancer where it has resulted in a virtual doubling of response rates compared to fluorouracil alone. By contrast methorexate acts by inhibiting folinic acid synthesis and so, following administration of high doses of the drug, any unacceptable toxicity can be arrested by giving intravenous or oral supplements of leucovorin.

Topoisomerase Inhibitors

Topoisomerase I and II are enzymes which help regulate DNA structure. Inhibition of these enzymes leads to single, or double, strand breakages in the DNA chain. The anthracycline drugs also act by intercalating with the DNA. This means that they sit within various parts of the DNA double helix, rather like a key in a lock, where their presence distorts the DNA template preventing the synthesis of nucleic acid.

The topoisomerase I inhibitors in general use are irinotecan and topotecan. The topoisomerase II inhibitors are etoposide, doxorubicin, epirubicin, idarubicin, daunorubicin, mitoxantrone and amsacrine. With the exception of etoposide and amsacrine, the topoisomerase II inhibitors listed here are also known as anthracyclines, or anthracycline antibiotics.

Cytotoxic Antibiotics

In 1940 the actinomycin antibiotics were first produced from cultures of the soil bacteria actinomycetes. Although actino-mycins did have antibacterial activity, they were considered too toxic for human use. Subsequent research produced Dacti-nomycin which proved to be an effective cytotoxic. Over the following decades a number of other cytotoxics were produced from bacterial cultures and became known collectively as cytotoxic antibiotics. As more became known about their precise modes of action, it became clear that some agents overlapped with other groups of cytotoxics, for example the anthracy-clines were also topoisomerase II inhibitors, pentostatin was an antimetabolite, and mitomycin had alkylating activity. Other cytotoxic antibiotics have different modes of action: dactino-mycin binds to DNA and prevents DNA transcription, it also causes DNA damage by free radical formation. Bleomycin also causes DNA fragmentation by free radical formation (free radicals are highly reactive molecules with unpaired electrons).

Anti-microtubule Drugs

In the past, infusions of the leaves of the garden periwinkle plant, *Vinca rosea*, were used in folk medicine as a treatment for diabetes. In the 1950s researchers in North America tested these infusions, looking for a hypoglycaemic action. Instead they discovered that the plant extracts caused leucopenia. Following these observations, two alkaloids were extracted from the periwinkle plant: vincristine and vinblastine, which have subse-quently proved to be valuable cytotoxic agents. Later vindesine and vinorelbine have been added to the family of vinca alkaloids.

In 1967 researchers in the United States, working on extracts of the bark of the Pacific yew tree, discovered the taxane cytotoxic paclitaxel. Subsequently a second, semi-synthetic taxane, docetaxel was produced, based on an extract of the needles of the European yew tree.

These drugs are all anti-microtubule cytotoxics. During the metaphase of mitosis, the daughter chromosomes are arranged on the cell spindle, before separating to form the two new cells. The cell spindle is formed by the protein tubulin. The anti-microtubule cytotoxics react with tubulin in one of two ways: the vinca alkaloids prevent the formation of the spindle and the taxanes stabilize, or freeze, the spindle so that the process of mitosis cannot proceed further. In both cases, cell death results. Because of their action on the spindle, these drugs are also often called cell spindle poisons.

A Note on Liposomal Formulations of Cytotoxic Drugs

Liposomes are spherical vesicles formed by a membrane made up of phospholipids and cholesterol. It is possible to encapsulate drugs within liposomes. In some instances the lipsomes may also be coated by polyethylene glycol (PEG), and this is known as a peglyated liposomal formulation. In the body the liposomal coating is broken down by enzymatic degradation, or attack by macrophages, to release the drug.

The possible advantages of this liposomal formulation for cytotoxic agents are that it might prolong their circulation time before they are metabolized or excreted, it might increase their entrapment in cancers, and may reduce their access to normal cells. These effects have the potential to increase the efficacy and reduce the toxicity of the drugs.

At present in the UK doxorubicin is the only liposomally formulated cytotoxic to have been licensed and is available in a liposomal and pegylated liposomal version. Both these formulations appear to offer a reduced risk of cardiotoxicity and cause less soft-tissue damage if the drug is extravagated; however hypersensitivity reactions and hand–foot syndrome (painful skin eruptions) are more common.

Liposomal formulations of the taxanes are also under evaluation. Both docetaxel and taxotere are difficult to get into solution and the additives necessary to do this are the agents responsible for the allergic reactions commonly seen with these agents. The liposomal formulation offers an alternative way of delivering these agents which may overcome the problem of hypersensitivity reactions for these drugs.

Suggestion for further reading
Park JW. Liposome-based drug delivery in breast cancer treatment. Breast Cancer Res, 2002; 4: 95–99.

The Development of Cytotoxic Therapy
Unlike many of the drugs that we have mentioned earlier in this chapter, cytotoxics have no ability to distinguish between cancer cells and normal cells. They will attack the process of cell division indiscriminately, and this causes many of their side effects, which are due to the direct damage of normal cells.

During the 1950s more cytotoxics became available, and it was realized that different drugs interfered with the process of cell division in different ways. The logical way forward was to combine drugs with different modes of action in order to maximize cell kill, by hitting the mitotic process from a number of different directions. The only problem was that this dramatically increased toxicity, because of the corresponding increase in damage to normal cells.

The solution came with a rescheduling of the way treatment was delivered. This took advantage of the fact that cancer cells, being biologically abnormal, are much slower than normal cells in repairing injury. Normal cells could make good the damage done by cytotoxics far more rapidly than cancer cells. Previously most cytotoxic treatments had been given continuously, and toxicity was dose-limiting. The breakthrough concept of the mid-1960s was to give the treatment intermittently (Fig. 1.9). So, if a high dose of a number of cytotoxics was given on a particular day (Day 1) then within 2 to 3 weeks the normal cells would have

(a)

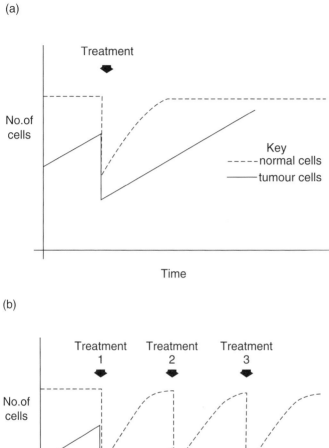

(b)

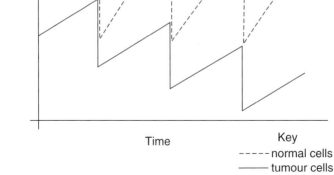

FIGURE 1.9. *Continued.*

(c)

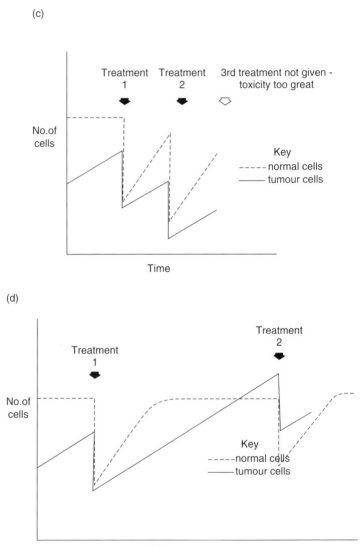

(d)

FIGURE 1.9. The rationale for intermittent courses of cytotoxic chemotherapy.
(**a**) After a course of cytotoxic chemotherapy normal and malignant cell numbers will be reduced, but because of their superior ability to repair injury the normal cells will recover more rapidly (**b**) by giving further courses of chemotherapy when normal cell recovery is

recovered but the cancer cells would still be struggling to repair the damage done. So if a second dose was given on, say, Day 21 or Day 28, normal cell recovery would be complete, but the cancer cells would be hit again before they had recovered, and so would be further damaged. By giving more courses, at the same interval, normal cell integrity could be maintained, whilst the cancer cells were progressively killed off. This is the principal of intermittent combination cytotoxic chemotherapy, and it under-pinned the great successes of cytotoxic therapy during the 1960s and 1970s.

Incidentally radiotherapy also works by interfering with mitosis (by forming free radicals which damage DNA in the nucleus). And, like cytotoxic therapy, ionizing radiations also cannot distinguish between normal and cancer cells. Once again the differences in repair capacity between normal and malignant cells come into play, but in this case radiation injury can be made good by normal cells in a matter of a few hours, rather than days or weeks, and so radiotherapy doses are usually given at daily intervals, rather than with the gap of several weeks needed for normal cell recovery with cytotoxic therapy.

Cytotoxic Drugs and the Cell Cycle
In the mid-1960s it was discovered that different cytotoxic drugs affected cells in the cell cycle in different ways (Fig. 1.10). Only one cytotoxic was found to affect cells in the resting Go stage (as well as all other phases of the cell cycle), this was nitrogen mustard. Many drugs were shown to attack cells at all phases of the active cell cycle. Because they only attacked cells which were actually in the cell cycle (as opposed to being in the resting Go stage), these were called cycle-specific drugs. They include cyclophosphamide, melphalan, chlorambucil, cispaltin, carboplatin, fluorouracil, mitomycin, doxorubicin, epirubicin and dacarbazine. Some other drugs only attacked cells during certain phases of the cell cycle. These were called cell cycle phase-specific drugs. They include methotrexate (active in S/early G1), cytarabine (S), vincristine (S), vinblastine (S) and bleomycin (G2/M).

FIGURE 1.9. complete, but before malignant cell numbers are restored the cancer can be destroyed with minimal damage to normal cell numbers. Timing is critical, however, because if the interval is too short unacceptable toxicity will result (**c**) whereas if it is too long the cancer will have the chance not only to recover but to actually increase in size (**d**).

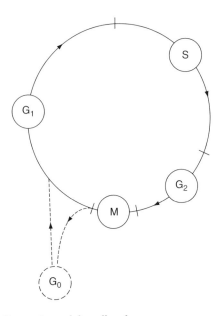

FIGURE 1.10. Cytotoxics and the cell cycle.
G_o are cells not actively dividing, G_1 is the first resting phase, S is the synthetic phase during which the cell's DNA content doubles, G_2 is the second resting, or pre-mitotic phase, and M is mitosis when the cell divides. Alkylating agents and platinum analogues act at all stages of the cell cycle except G_o. Antimetabolites and topoisomerase inhibitors act mainly during the S phase. Antibiotics work mainly during G_2 and M. Spindle cell poisons work during the M phase.

During the 1970s oncologists tried to exploit these differences by designing drug combinations and treatment schedules based on cell cycle theory. At the end of the day clinical trials showed absolutely no benefit from these complex drug regimens, and they fell out of favour. These days little or no attention is paid to cell cycle kinetics in the design of drug combinations and treatment schedules. So this whole question is really only of historic interest.

TUMOUR KINETICS: ADJUVANT THERAPY

With the start of uncontrolled mitosis the cancer has now begun to grow. In the 1960s Howard Skipper, working in Alabama, discovered that injecting a single leukaemic cell into an immune-suppressed mouse could lead to a fatal leukaemia, showing that cancerous changes in just one cell were sufficient to be lethal. So, one cell divides to become two, two divide to become four, and so on.

After some 20 cell divisions, or cell doublings, our cancer will contain about 100 million cells, and form a swelling approximately 0.5cm in diameter (Fig. 1.11). This is about the smallest size at which most cancers can be detected clinically, by physical examination or radiological imaging. After about another 20 doublings the cancer will have achieved a lethal tumour burden and the host will die.

Although tumour growth tends to slow with time, as the intervals between doublings gradually increases, these figures still mean that for a large part of its natural history a cancer will be completely clinically undetectable: tumour masses containing hundreds of millions of cancer cells may be present that will not be revealed by the even the most careful examination or the most detailed CT or MRI scans.

This explains why someone can have an operation to remove a primary cancer, and appear to be free of all traces of the disease, yet still relapse with widespread secondary disease, with multiple bone, or liver, or lung metastases, a matter of months or years later. Those secondary cancers did not develop after the primary

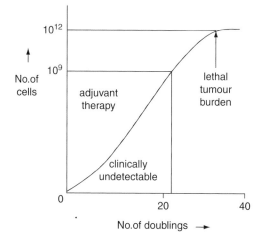

FIGURE 1.11. Tumour cell population and the limit of clinical detection
As the tumour grows its growth rate slows as it begins to outgrow its blood supply and more cells move into the G_o phase of the cell cycle.

was removed, they were there at the time of the original operation, but were simply too small to be detectable.

In the 1960s this appreciation of basic tumour kinetics coincided with the major improvements in treatment of a number of advanced, metastatic, cancers as result of intermittent combination cytotoxic chemotherapy. As a result a number of experts put forward a new concept: if cytotoxic chemotherapy could reduce large tumour volumes might it not be even more effective against small, microscopic foci of cancer, so that if one could identify patients who were at risk of harbouring these occult metastases after surgery for a primary cancer, and if one gave them chemotherapy, could that then kill off those potentially lethal secondary cancers, and cure them?

This was put to the test in breast cancer. The presence of cancer in one or more of the axillary lymph nodes was taken as an indicator that there was a risk of spread elsewhere in the body, and clinical trails were established where women who had node-positive disease were randomized to receive either no further treatment or systemic therapy, with either cytotoxic drugs or hormonal agents. These trials rapidly showed that giving drug treatment dramatically reduced relapse rates and improved overall survival. The case for introducing systemic therapy for selected patients in the treatment of the early stages of breast cancer was proven.

This approach of giving treatment to patients who are at risk of harbouring microscopic metastases after their primary treatment, even though they have no clinical evidence of disease, is called adjuvant therapy. Over the last 30 years, following the pioneering work in breast cancer, adjuvant therapy now forms a routine part of the management of a number of major cancers.

Although the introduction of adjuvant therapy has improved the outcomes in a number of cancers, it is important to remember that this is a treatment of a risk, not a certainty. As the residual cancer that is being treated is, by definition, undetectable, it is impossible to know whether it is there or not, all one can say is that because of the features of their primary cancer that particular individual has a *probability* of still harbouring occult metastases. This means that in any group of individuals given adjuvant treatment a number will already have been cured by their initial surgery, or radiotherapy, and will be receiving their systemic therapy completely unnecessarily.

A further point about adjuvant therapy, which many patients find hard to understand, is that because there is no detectable or measurable disease at the outset, then there is no short-term way of knowing whether or not the treatment has worked. Doing scans, x-rays or blood tests at the end of systemic adjuvant therapy won't give the answer, and the only way of knowing if treatment has been successful is if the patient is alive and disease-free some 5 to 10 years later.

GENE ANALYSIS AND TREATMENT SELECTION

Historically progress in systemic cancer therapy has come from the discovery of new drugs, or developing new ways of exploiting existing therapies. The problems of patient selection, touched on in the previous section on adjuvant therapy, have been largely overlooked but are now coming into sharper focus. Unlike antibiotic therapy, where laboratory testing can be done to identify the appropriate drug treatment, no 'culture and sensitivity' test has ever been successfully developed for cancers (despite countless attempts to do so). However, developments in technology based around gene analysis are offering the possibility that this may soon change.

In recent years laboratory methods have been developed that allow tissue samples to be rapidly analysed for the presence of thousands of different genes. The two techniques used to do this are called DNA microassay (or gene array assay) and real-time reverse transcriptase polymerase chain reaction (RT-RTPCR) analysis.

Cancers are made up of abnormal cells and these cells contain abnormal patterns of genes. Even with the same type of cancer different patients will have different patterns of abnormal genes in their cancer cells.

It has always been recognized that individual cancers can behave quite differently. For example, two women may both have early breast cancer, and their tumours may look very similar under the microscope, but one might be growing very aggressively and spreading rapidly, whilst the other might grow much more slowly.

The way these different cancers behave is controlled by their genes. Research using gene expression profiling is currently being used to study cancers to see if a high-risk gene signature can be identified. This is a particular pattern of abnormal genes which means that the particular cancer is likely to behave more aggressively.

Some progress has been made in breast cancer and lung cancer in discovering high-risk gene signatures. But this process is still at an early stage of development and gene expression profiling is still very much at the research stage.

The hope is that in years to come it may be a more routine process and may not only help in deciding whether a cancer is more or less aggressive, but might actually help in deciding what the best treatment for that cancer might be.

Suggestions for further reading

Chen H-Y, Yu S-L, Chen C-H, et al. A five-gene signature and clinical outcome in non-small-cell lung cancer. New Engl J Med, 2007; 356: 11–20.

Fan C, Oh DS, Wessels L, et al. Concordance among gene-expression based predictors for breast cancer. New Engl J Med, 2006; 355: 560–569.

BISPHOSPHONATES

Although there is some laboratory evidence that the bisphosphonates may have a direct effect on cancer cells, their main role in oncology is as a supportive therapy. They alter bone metabolism, their net effect being inhibition of osteoclast activity, leading to a reduction in bone resorption, and hence bone strengthening. This has led to their evaluation in people who have, or are at risk of developing, skeletal involvement from their cancer.

Bisphosphonates have been most extensively studied in multiple myeloma, breast and prostate cancer. In people with multiple myeloma, and those with bone secondaries from breast or prostate cancer, clinical trials show that bisphosphonates reduce the risk of pathological fractures and malignant hypercalcaemia. The need for palliative radiotherapy and orthopaedic surgery is also reduced, but the risk of spinal cord compression is not affected. In multiple myeloma there is clear evidence that bisphosphonates also help with pain control, but this is less certain in breast and prostate cancer. Despite these various benefits the use of bisphosphonates does not improve overall survival in any of these patient groups.

At the present time bisphosphonates do form part of the routine management of patients with multiple myeloma (except for those with the indolent, or smouldering, from of the disease). The extent to which they are used in people who have bone secondaries from breast or prostate cancer is variable, but increasing. Some clinical trials have also suggested that bisphosphonates may have a role in adjuvant therapy for early breast cancer, reducing the risk of bone involvement but, in the UK at least, they are not routinely used in this indication.

Bisphosphonates are available in oral and intravenous formulations (Table 1.8). The optimum duration of bisphosphonate therapy has still to be defined, but the usual practice is for the

TABLE 1.8. Bisphosphonates used in cancer care

Drug	Formulation
Disodium pamidronate	Intravenous
Ibandronic acid	Oral
Sodium clodronate	Oral
Zoledronic acid	Intravenous

drugs to be given until there is clear evidence that they are no longer effective. The complications include gastrointestinal disturbance (nausea, diarrhoea or constipation) which is more likely with oral farmulations, fevers, and hypocalcaemia, which are more likely with intravenous therapy. An uncommon, but severe, complication is osteonecrosis of the jaw. This affects between 1% and 5% of patients receiving intravenous zoledronic acid or pamidronate for more than 18 months; it is more likely in people with pre-existing dental problems or those requiring major dental work during treatment.

Suggestion for further reading
Bilezikian JP. Osteonecrosis of the jaw – do bisphosphonates pose a risk? N Engl J Med, 2006; 355: 2278–2281.

Body J-J. Bisphosphonates for malignancy-related bone disease: current status, future developments. Supp Care Cancer, 2006; 14: 408–418.

Ross JR, Saunders Y, Edmonds PM et al. Systematic review of role of bisphosphonates on skeletal morbidity in metastatic cancer. Br Med J, 2003: 327: 469–472.

CHEMOPREVENTION

To bring this chapter full circle it is reasonable to pose the following question: If drugs can be used to treat cancer can they also be used to prevent it? As far as the cytotoxics are concerned, side effects preclude their use in this situation but hormonal approaches have been explored in breast and prostate cancer.

A number of clinical trials have been carried out randomizing women who have been assessed on the basis of their family history as being at high risk of developing breast cancer to receive either tamoxifen or a placebo. The results of individual trials differ but a meta-analysis has revealed that giving tamoxifen reduces the overall risk of breast cancer development by up to 40%. Despite this apparent good news there are some uncertainties about these results: the risk reduction applies only to ER+ cancers, and the women are exposed to the side effects of tamoxifen, including an increased risk of thromboembolic phenomena and endometrial cancer, furthermore no study has yet shown an overall increase in survival as a result of giving tamoxifen. Different parts of the world have reached different conclusions about these results: in the United States guidelines have been formulated for the use of tamoxifen in breast cancer prevention whereas in UK no such recommendations have been made.

More recent trials in breast cancer chemoprevention have focused on a number of other alternatives, including tamoxifen in low doses and raloxifene – a selective oestrogen receptor modifier used to treat osteoporosis, but not breast cancer, which may be as effective as tamoxifen but without some of its side effects, including the risk of endometrial cancer – and evaluating the use of aromatase inhibitors. Unlike tamoxifen, which appears equally effective at all ages, the aromatase inhibitors would only be suitable for post-menopausal women.

In prostate cancer one large study has looked at giving volunteers the drug finasteride on a daily basis for 7 years and shown a 25% reduction in the incidence of the disease. Finasteride inhibits the enzyme 5α-reductase which is involved in testosterone metabolism and hence reduces circulating androgen levels, and it is usually used in benign prostatic hypertrophy where it leads to shrinkage of the gland and relief of obstructive symptoms. Once again, although this study did show promising results there were problems in that side effects such as impotence, loss of libido and breast enlargement were troublesome, and there was a greater incidence of big-grade, more aggressive, prostate cancers among the men who took the drug. Consequently finasteride is not currently recommended for prostate cancer prophylaxis.

Despite these mixed results the subject of chemoprevention remains a very active research area, and the newer forms of anti-cancer agents, such as the vascular and epidermal growth receptor inhibitors and tyrosine kinase inhibitors, may offer other opportunities for studies in the future.

Suggestions for further reading
Gasco M, Argusti A, Bonanni B, Decensi A. SERMs in chemoprevention of breast cancer. Eur J Cancer, 2005; 41: 1980–1989.

O'Regan RM. Breast cancer chemoprevention. Lancet, 2005; 366: 1506–1508.

Mellon JK. The finasteride prostate cancer prevention trial (PCPT) – what have we learned? Eur J Cancer, 2005; 2016–2022.

Part 2
Some Practical Aspects of Cancer Chemotherapy

DRUG DOSING

For the last 50 years most cytotoxics have been prescribed in relation to the patient's body surface area. The surface area is calculated from their height and weight, either by the use of nomograms or pre-programmed calculators or computers. The same principle is used for some, but not all, of the newer targeted therapies but, by contrast, hormonal treatments are almost always prescribed in standard doses that are the same for everybody.

The original rationale for prescribing cytotoxics on the basis of body surface area came from the realization that there was only a narrow therapeutic window between unacceptable toxicity and efficacy for many of these agents: give too large a dose and the patient could well die from side effects, give too small a dose and the drug would be ineffective against the cancer, and often the margin for error would be small. So there was a need to individualize cytotoxic dosing. Many different factors may influence someone's response to a given dose of a drug, including their age, sex, their body size, any co-morbidities, liver and kidney function which might affect drug metabolism and excretion, and other drugs they are receiving. Measuring and assessing all these parameters for every patient is not generally practical and research in the late 1950s indicated that, for cytotoxics, adjusting the dose of drug according to the patient's surface area was an acceptable surrogate in most instances. So the convention was established of prescribing cytotoxics on the basis of Xmg/m^2 surface area.

One cytotoxic that is the exception to this rule is carboplatin. The toxicity of carboplatin is closely related to its concentration in the blood over time, which in turn relates to its clearance by the kidney. The dose of carboplatin is therefore worked out by a formula, the Calvert formula, which takes account of a target blood/time level (the area under the curve, or AUC) and renal function (in terms of the glomerular filtration rate, GFR). The target AUC is usually either 5 or 7mg/ml per minute (depending on whether the patient has had previous treatment or not). The GFR may either be measured directly by the ^{51}Cr-EDTA method or calculated by formulae such as those of Cockroft-Gault, Jellieff or Chatelet, based on measurements of serum creatinine. The Calvert formula is dose = AUC × (GFR + 25).

Suggestions for further reading

Gurney H. Developing a new framework for dose calculation. J Clin Oncol 2006; 24: 1489–1490.

Kaestner SA, Sewell GJ. Chemotherapy dosing part I: scientific basis for current practice and use of body surface area. Clin Oncol 2007; 19: 23–37.

Kaestner SA, Sewell GJ. Chemotherapy dosing part II: alternative approaches and future prospects. Clin Oncol 2007; 19: 99–107.

DRUG DELIVERY

Venous Lines

Historically, having a course of chemotherapy involved multiple venepunctures, both for all the blood tests that needed to be done and for giving the drugs themselves. This had disadvantages from a patient's point of view – repeated discomfort, needle phobia – and practically: the difficulty of finding 'a good vein'. Increasingly nowadays using a venous line offers an alternative. The line is a fine hollow silicone rubber catheter, which is inserted into a vein, and stays in place throughout the time of the chemotherapy. Two types of line are used: a central line or a PICC (peripherally inserted central catheter) line. Central lines are also sometimes known by the names of the manufacturers of the lines, the two main ones being Hickman and Groshong.

The central line is inserted through the skin just below the collar bone. It is then tunnelled for a distance subcutaneously before entering into the subclavian vein, and then threaded through this until its tip lies in the superior vena cava, just above the heart (Photo 1). The subcutaneous tunnelling of the line helps reduce the risk of infection in the line. A PICC line is inserted through one of the large veins near the bend of the elbow, and threaded along this, through the subclavian vein and into the superior vena cava.

PICC lines are cheaper and simpler to insert than central lines but are usually only suitable for short-term therapies over a maximum of 6–8 weeks, whereas central lines can stay in place

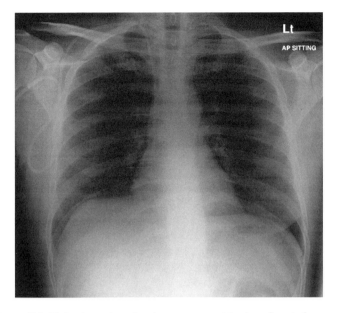

PHOTO 2.1. Plain chest x-ray showing correct positioning of central venous line (courtesy of Mr Anthony Leese, New Cross Hospital, Wolverhampton)

for a year or more. Also many oncologists feel that drugs which are likely to cause irritation to the veins, such as anthracycline cytotoxics (doxorubicin and epirubicin) and fluorouracil, are not suitable for use with PICC lines.

Once in place, the line can be used for taking blood tests, and for giving all the drugs that would normally have to be injected into a vein, or given through a drip. Putting in the line is a simple procedure. Placing a PICC line can be done as an out-patient and does not need a general anaesthetic. The skin where the line is to be inserted is numbed with local anaesthetic, and threading the line through the veins is usually quite painless, so there should not be much discomfort while this is being done. The insertion only takes a few minutes and is followed immediately by a chest x-ray to check that the tip of the line is in the correct position. Putting in a central line is very similar, but sometimes this may be done with a short general anaesthetic rather than a local anaesthetic.

Once the line is in place it is important that it does not get blocked. To prevent this it will have to be flushed through on a regular basis. Typical schedules for this are a weekly flush with 50iu of heparin in 5ml of 0.9% saline once weekly, or 500iu heparin in 5ml saline once monthly, or simply regular flushes with saline. This may be done by chemotherapy nurses or by the patients themselves.

Normally lines are relatively trouble-free. The most common problems that do occur are shown in Table 2.1. Of the immediate problems, which occur at the time of line insertion, the arrhythmias although the commonest are not usually clinically significant. The reported incidence of late complications varies enormously in different series. When thrombosis occurs it may be of one of three types:

1. Fibrin sheath formation around the catheter: this is only troublesome if it affects the tip of the catheter, leading to complete or partial obstruction.
2. Intraluminal thrombosis: this may either go undetected or may lead to blockage of the catheter.
3. Blood vessel thrombosis: effectively a deep vein thrombosis in the vessel around the catheter.

Apart from possible catheter obstruction thrombosis may lead to pulmonary embolism, which complicates 5% of thrombotic episodes, or the associated phlebitis may result in venous distension and swelling of the ipsilateral arm, which may complicate up to 10% of thromboses.

Removing lines is usually very simple. It is done in the out-patient clinic, with just a local anaesthetic to avoid any discomfort, and only takes a few minutes.

TABLE 2.1. Complications of central venous line insertion

Immediate – at the time of insertion	
Cardiac arrhythmia	13%
Arterial puncture	2%
Tip in wrong position	2%
Pneumothorax	1%
Haemorrhage	1%
Late – following insertion	
Infection	4–40%
Thrombosis	
Symptomatic	5–40%
Asymptomatic	5–60%
Migration of catheter tip	5%
Fracture of catheter	3%

% indicates the frequency of these complications, but their incidence varies widely in different series.

Suggestions for further reading

British Committee for Standards in Haematology. BCSH guidelines on the insertion and management of central venous access devices in adults, 2006. www.bcshguidelines.com.

Rosovsky RP, Kuter DJ. Central venous catheters: care and complications. In Chabner BA, Longo DL eds. Cancer chemotherapy and biotherapy, 4th edition. Lippincott, Williams and Wilkins, 2006, pp. 516–528.

Implantable Ports

Implantable ports (which are also known as portocaths) are a variation on venous lines. The line is placed in a similar way, but instead of the end of it coming out on the skin, it ends in a subcutaneous port. This is a small soft plastic bubble, between about 2.5 and 4 cm across, which lies just under the surface of the skin. This means it is less obvious than a central or PICC line, and appears as just a small bump under the skin. It is usually placed near the top of the front of the chest.

Like central lines, implantable ports may be inserted either as an out-patient, using a local anaesthetic, or occasionally as a day-patient, if a general anaesthetic is used. They also need regular flushing to stop them becoming blocked.

Once in place implantable ports can be used just like the venous lines: for taking blood tests, or giving chemotherapy or blood transfusions or other intravenous fluids.

INFUSION PUMPS

When a chemotherapy drug is given into a vein it is usual to set up an intravenous infusion, with a bag of fluid, on a drip stand, which trickles through a tube into the vein. The drug may either be given as an injection into the tubing of the drip, or it may be mixed with the fluid in the bag and run in as an infusion.

Depending on the treatment that is being given, the infusion may last for anywhere from a few minutes to a few hours. But some chemotherapy treatments require the drugs to be given into a vein over a matter of days or even weeks. For these long infusions, a portable pump can be used, along with a venous line. The pump may be either a battery driven device that holds a syringe containing the chemotherapy drug (Photo 2), or a disposable vacuum operated device, an elastomeric pump (Photo 3). This is attached to the end of the venous line, and very slowly the pump squeezes a trickle of the drug into the vein. Once the infusion is complete, then the pump is easily disconnected.

Pumps vary in size, but are usually little bigger than a mobile phone. They can be worn in a special 'holster', meaning that they

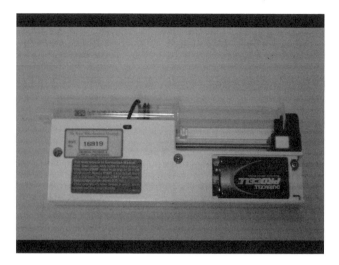

PHOTO 2.2. A battery-driven chemotherapy pump (courtesy of Mr Simon Glazebrook, New Cross Hospital Wolverhampton) (*See* Color plate 1)

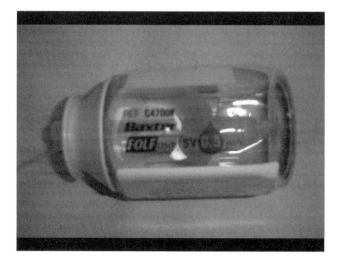

PHOTO 2.3. A disposable elastomeric infusion pump (courtesy of Mr Simon Glazebrook, New Cross Hospital Wolverhampton) (*See* Color plate 2)

are easy to carry around, and not very obvious. This means that treatment can continue when the patient is at home, and there should be very little effect on their normal day-to-day activities while the infusion is in progress.

Epidural Chemotherapy
Very occasionally, most often with certain types of leukaemia, it may be necessary to give chemotherapy drugs via a lumbar puncture, into the space around the spinal cord, so that the drug can reach parts of the nervous system that it might not get to if it was given by an ordinary infusion into a vein. This type of treatment is called epidural chemotherapy. Unfortunately in the UK there have been a number of fatal accidents in the past as a result of this technique –when either the wrong drug or wrong doses of a cytotoxic were given. Because of this there are now very strict regulations and protocols governing this particular type of treatment.

SIDE EFFECTS OF CANCER CHEMOTHERAPY
Most chemotherapy today is still based on the use of cytotoxic drugs; hormonal treatment is important in breast and prostate cancer, and the newer targeted therapies are gaining an increasing role in cancer treatment. These different groups of drugs have very different patterns of toxicity. Because of the frequency and potential severity of their side effects, the potential adverse reactions to cytotoxics will be considered in some detail in this section. While discussing these, it is important to remember that patients often react differently to the same treatment. Two people can have identical chemotherapy, for the same type of cancer, and be of similar age, with a similar level of fitness, one may experience virtually no problems, whilst the other might suffer considerable side effects, and their treatment may be quite challenging.

Common Side Effects of Cytotoxic Treatment
Cytotoxic drugs interfere directly with the process of mitosis. They have no ability to distinguish between cancer cells and normal cells, and so inhibit cell division in both populations. This accounts for many of their side effects. This means that the use of cytotoxic treatment is the art of differential poisoning: killing the cancer without killing the patient. Unfortunately it is easy to get this balance wrong and people still regularly die from the side effects of cytotoxic chemotherapy. Being aware of what those side

effects are, and being vigilant to detect their development as early as possible, is therefore a priority for all clinicians involved with this form of treatment.

There are many different cytotoxic drugs, and many different combinations of these drugs are used in cancer treatment. This means that the potential side effects vary considerably depending on the drugs, and the doses that are used. Having said this, there are some side effects that occur much more often than others. These include bone marrow suppression, nausea and vomiting, tiredness, alopecia, oral mucositis, reduced fertility and the risk of second cancers.

Marrow Suppression

Normally the effect of a dose of chemotherapy on the bone marrow cells is temporary. The changes come on a few days after treatment, reaching a peak at about 10–14 days, and then recovering over the next week or so.

The production of white blood cells is the process most sensitive to cytotoxic inhibition; changes to the red cells, and platelets, generally occur more slowly and are only likely to show up after several courses of chemotherapy (and very often are not affected at all, throughout the entire treatment). Typically the white cell count begins to fall at about 5–7 days after a dose of cytotoxics and will reach its lowest level about 2 weeks after the treatment. The count then recovers and will be more or less back to normal by the end of the third week. This means that there is an increased risk of infection while having chemotherapy. The combination of an infection with neutropenia is termed neutropenic sepsis. This is a common and serious complication. In those patients who require hospitalization, who make up the great majority, the mortality rate may be as high as 10%, being slightly greater for those with haematological malignancies and slightly lower for people with solid cancers.

There is no universally agreed definition of neutropenic sepsis, many centres use a body temperature $>38^oC$ and a neutrophil count $<1 \times 10^9$/L as their defining criteria, whereas others use a temperature $>38.5^oC$ and a neutrophil count $<0.5 \times 10^9$/L.

The risk and severity of infection is highest in people with profound neutropenia ($<0.1 \times 10^9$/L) or with neutropenia lasting >14 days. Patients with haematologic malignancies or those patients receiving high-dose chemotherapy are at the highest risk of neutropenic sepsis as they often have a neutrophil count $\leq 0.1 \times 10^9$/L for more than 14 days. Patients receiving conventional chemotherapy for solid malignancy usually have a period of neutropenia lasting for a period of 7–10 days. Therefore, neutropenia in these patients has a much lower risk. Some chemotherapy regimens are more likely than others to cause profound neutropenia (Table 2.2). Other factors which increase risk of infections in these patients include damage to the skin or gastrointestinal mucosa, the use of central lines, their nutritional status and general fitness.

The degree of risk should be assessed in advance for individual patients. They should then be warned of that risk, and the usual advice would be that if, at any time during treatment, they get a temperature of more than 38°C (100.5°F), or if they develop symptoms suggesting an infection – like shivering, a sore throat,

TABLE 2.2. Chemotherapy regimens associated with A greater than 20% risk of febrile neutropenia

Acronym	Drugs	Indication
AT	doxorubicin, docetaxel	Breast cancer
CAV	cyclophosphamide, doxorubicin, vincristine	Lung cancer
DHAP	dexamethasone, cisplatin, cytarabine	Non-Hodgkin's lymphoma
Doc	docetaxel	Breast cancer
ESHAP	etoposide, methylprednisolone, cisplatin, cytarabine	Non-Hodgkin's lymphoma
TAC	docetaxel, doxorubicin, cyclophosphamide	Breast cancer
Topo	topotecan	Lung cancer
VAPEC-B	vincristine, doxorubicin, prednisolone, etoposide, cyclophosphamide, bleomycin	Non-Hodgkin's lymhpoma
VelP	vinblastine, ifosfamide cisplatin	Germ cell (testicular cancer)

or a cough and shortness of breath, or cystitis, or if they simply suddenly feel unwell – then they should let the hospital know immediately, so that they can attend for assessment.

Neutropenic sepsis has usually been considered a medical emergency requiring admission to hospital and treatment with intensive intravenous antibiotic therapy. It is now recognized, however, that in some cases the condition can be managed more conservatively, with oral antibiotics being given on an out-patient basis. The advantages of out-patient therapy include fewer super-infections caused by hospital acquired infections, greater convenience for the patient, more efficient use of resources and reduced costs. This approach is most likely to be possible for people with solid tumours. There are no universally agreed criteria for deciding who can or cannot be managed in this way, but Table 2.3 sets out some general guidelines.

The antibiotics used, the doses given and the duration of treatment vary from hospital to hospital, for both in-patient and out-patient management of neutropenic sepsis. Every unit that delivers cytotoxic therapy will have a policy in place for the management of neutropenic sepsis that will specify their local regimens.

Wherever possible once someone has recovered from an episode of neutropenic sepsis the aim will be for them to continue their planned chemotherapy with no dose reduction. For some people this may involve the use of prophylactic antibiotics prior

TABLE 2.3. Possible criteria for defining patients with neutropenic sepsis who may be managed on an out-patient basis

All of the following criteria must be met

1. Solid tumour malignancy
2. Absolute neutrophil count $> 0.1 \times 10^9/L$
3. Good performance status
4. Expected duration of neutropenia less than 7 days
5. Their cancer is controlled (mild symptoms only)
6. No other significant comorbid condition
7. No hypotension
8. No dehydration
9. Age < 70
10. No evidence of indwelling central–line infection
11. No antibiotic therapy in the previous 96 hours (including prophylactic antibiotics)
12. Patient able to manage oral tablet therapy–minimal or no dysphagia or mucositis
13. Patient likely to comply with oral therapy
14. Patient not at home alone

to and during subsequent cycles of treatment, for others the use of granulocyte colony stimulating factors (GCSF) may be considered. Once again the guidelines for using GCSF vary from country to country (in part influenced by cost considerations) and

TABLE 2.4. Typical UK indications for the use of GSCF in patients receiving cytotoxic chemotherapy

GCSF may be used as either primary prophylaxis, to prevent the development of severe neutropenia, or secondary prophylaxis, to prevent recurrence of neutropenia with subsequent courses of treatment after an initial episode of neutropenic sepsis. It may also be used therapeutically in the management of neutropenic sepsis.

1. Primary prophylaxis

Primary prophylaxis may be considered in the following circumstances:

  i) Patients receiving radical or adjuvant chemotherapy who are at ≥ 40% risk of developing neutropenic fever
  ii) Hospitalized patients receiving radical or adjuvant chemotherapy who are at ≥ 20% risk of developing neutropenic fever while an in-patient.
  iii) Patients aged > 65 receiving radical or adjuvant chemotherapy who are at ≥ 20% risk of developing neutropenic fever
  iv) Patients aged >50 with significant pulmonary or cardiovascular comorbidity receiving radical or adjuvant chemotherapy who are at ≥ 20% risk of developing neutropenic fever
  v) Patients aged with leukaemia or lymphoma receiving radical chemotherapy who are at ≥ 20% risk of developing neutropenic fever

The risk is assessed on the basis of the patient's age, tumour type, performance status, comorbidities and the likely myelotoxicity of the chosen drug regimen (see Table 2.2).

2. Secondary prophylaxis.
The use of GCSF should be considered in patients receiving curative chemotherapy for cancers where maintenance of dose intensity may improve survival. However the optimum scheduling of GCSF is not defined.

3. Therapeutic use

  i) Prolonged neutropenia (neutrophil count <1.0 × 10^9/L) after chemotherapy for more than 7 days
  ii) Chronic cyclical neutropenia with severe neutropenia and recurrent infections
  iii) Profound or severe neutropenia (neutrophil count <0.5) in patients with factors predisposing to a high risk of infection such as severe mucositis or enteritis

from department to department, but Table 2.4 gives a typical set of criteria in the UK.

The incidence of anaemia during chemotherapy, defined by haemoglobin (Hb) level of <10g/dl, is difficult to quantify, with estimates ranging from 20% to 60% of patients being affected. Clearly when the Hb level does fall below 10g/dl symptoms will usually be fairly obvious, and treatment can be given. In the last few years, however, a number of studies have shown that patients can experience fatigue and other symptoms, when their Hb level falls to between 10 and 12g/dl during their treatment. This is a level that many clinicians would not usually consider as significantly anaemic but treatment to bring their Hb to above the 12g/dl level has been shown to greatly improve their quality of life. The choice of treatment rests between blood transfusion and the use of erythropoietic agents such as epoetin alfa, or darbepoietin alfa, to stimulate red blood cell production. The latter are effective, but expensive when compared to transfusions. In the USA previous guidelines suggest transfusion if an immediate correction of anaemia is necessary, but recommend erythropoietic agents for symptomatic patients with an Hb level below 11g/dl during their chemotherapy. There are no equivalent guidelines in the UK. However, the results from some recent studies have raised questions over the safety of these agents, suggesting they could lead to an increase in cancer growth and might cause thromboembolic complications. The evidence for these concerns is currently being reviewed by the drug safety authorities, and it is likely that new guidance will follow in due course.

Suggestion for further reading

Ferrario E, Ferrari L, Bidoli P et al. Treatment of cancer-related anemia with epoietin alfa: a review. Cancer Treat Rev, 2005; 30: 563–575.

Pagliuca A, Carrington PA, Pettengell R et al. Guidelines for the use of colony stimulating factors in haematological malignancy. Br J Haemtol, 2004; 123: 22–33.

Smith TJ, Khatcheresian J, Lyman GH et al. 2006 update of recommendations for the use of white blood cell growth factors: an evidence-based clinical practice guideline. J Clin Oncol, 2006; 24: 3187–3205.

Steensma DP. Erythropoiesis stimulating agents may not be safe in people with cancer. Br Med J, 2007; 334: 648–649.

Nausea and Vomiting

Many cytotoxic treatments result in nausea and vomiting. The nausea comes on a few hours after the drugs are given. It is usually at its worst during the first 2 days after the chemotherapy, and then settles quite quickly over another day or two. The chance of experiencing sickness, and its severity, varies enormously with different cytotoxic drugs, and the commonly used agents may be classified into those at high risk of emesis (where >90% of patients are likely to be affected), moderate risk (30 to 90%), low risk (10 to 30%) and minimal risk (<10%) (Table 2.5). There is also evidence that some people are more vulnerable to chemotherapy-

TABLE 2.5. The emetic potential of anti-cancer drugs

Minimal risk

Alpha interferon	Imatinib
Bevacizumab	Melphalan oral
Bleomycin	Mercaptopurine
Busulfan	Methotrexate <50mg/m^2
Cetuximab	Pentostatin
Chlorambucil	Rituximab
Cladribine	Vinblastine
Fludarabine	Vincristine
Gefitinib	Vindesine
Hydroxyurea	Vinorelbine

Low risk

Bortezomib	Mitomycin
Capecitabine	Mitoxantrone
Cytaribine <200mg/m^2	Paclitaxel
Docetaxel	Pemetrexed
Etoposide	Thioguanine
Fluorouracil <1G/m^2	Topotecan
Gemcitabine	Trastuzumab
Methotrexate >50mg/m^2	

Moderate risk

Amsacrine	Idarubicin
Carboplatin	Ifosfamide
Carmustine <250mg/m^2	Interleukin
Cisplatin <70mg/m^2	Irinotecan
Cyclophosphamide <1500mg/m^2	Lomustine
Cytarabine >1000mg/m^2	Melpahalan iv
Daunorubicin	Oxaliplatin
Doxorubicin	Procarbazine
Epirubicin	Temozolamide
Fluorouracil > 1000mg/m^2	

High risk

Carmustine >250mg/m^2	Dacarbazine
Cisplatin >70mg/m^2	Dactinomycin
Cyclophosphamide >1500mg/m^2	Nitrogen mustard

induced nausea and vomiting than others: women are more at risk than men, especially if they have experienced emesis during pregnancy; younger people are more at risk than older people; and a history of motion sickness means problems are more likely. A key point in managing cytotoxic emesis is to prevent it happening in the first place, so anti-emetic treatment is usually given as prophylaxis, rather than waiting for symptoms to develop.

For many years control of emesis relied on dopamine antagonists like metoclopramide (Maxolon) or domperidone (Motilium). Prevention and treatment of cytotoxic-induced emesis then improved dramatically in the 1990s with the introduction of the 5HT3 receptor antagonists, ondansetron (Zofran) or granisetron (Kytril). 5HT3 receptors, which are stimulated by serotonin (5-hydroxytryptamine), form part of both the central and the peripheral pathways for the stimulation of nausea and vomiting. The effectiveness of all these drugs can be further increased by giving the steroid, dexamethasone, which is an effective anti-emetic in its own right, at the same time. A recent development is the introduction of a drug called aprepitant (Emend). This works in a different way to other anti-sickness drugs by inhibiting neurokinin-1 (NK_1) receptors in the brain. These receptors are key to triggering the vomiting reflex, they are stimulated by a neurotransmitter called substance P. Aprepitant seems particularly good at preventing the delayed sickness that comes on a day or two after treatment, which is a particular feature of some drugs, especially cisplatin.

The protocol for anti-emetic therapy can be tailored to the risk of symptoms developing. So for minimal risk drugs treatment may not be necessary but if problems do occur then metoclopramide or domperidone, starting immediately prior to chemotherapy and given tds for 4 days, should suffice. For low-risk therapy a single dose of 8mg dexamethasone 30–60 minutes before drug administration is recommended. For moderate risk drugs a single dose of dexamethasone, either orally or iv, together with a 5HT3 antagonist, orally or iv, immediately prior to treatment should be followed by an oral 5HT3 antagonist for the next 72 hours. A similar regimen may be used for high-risk drugs, but aprepitant may be added to the schedule if necessary. These schedules will prevent sickness altogether, or keep it to a very low, and tolerable, level for the great majority of people.

Incidentally, although 5HT3 antagonists are very effective at preventing and relieving sickness, some people do find they get side effects from them. The most common of these are consti-

TABLE 2.6. Advice for patients to reduce their risk of nausea

- Avoid greasy, fatty or very spicy foods
- Ginger can help to ease sickness so try nibbling a ginger biscuit or drinking ginger ale or ginger beer
- Avoid big meals, eat little and often with light bites and snacks
- If you feel sick first thing in the morning, keep a couple of dry biscuits by your bed and try to eat one before you get up
- Make sure you have plenty of fresh air; keep a window open if you can, especially when cooking
- If cooking smells upset you, try to get someone else to prepare your meals, or opt for cold food, with salads and sandwiches
- Sea-bands may be helpful. These are bands that you strap on round your wrists. They are fitted with a button that gently presses on the skin over an acupressure point on the inner surface of the wrist. You can buy these sea-bands from any chemists

pation and headache. These can usually be relieved with a simple laxative like Senokot, or a simple painkiller like paracetemol.

In addition to these pharmacological measures, there are also things that patients can do themselves to help reduce the risk of nausea during chemotherapy. These are summarized in Table 2.6.

Suggestion for further reading
Kris MG, Hesketh PJ, Somerfield MR et al. American Society of Clinical Oncology guidelines for antiemetics in oncology: update 2006. J Clin Oncol, 2006; 24: 2932–2947.

Tiredness or Fatigue
Profound tiredness, or fatigue, is a very common problem during chemotherapy. It is thought that four out of five people will experience fatigue on some days during their treatment, and for about one in three it will be present most of the time. Not only is there often a complete lack of energy, but the tiredness can also interfere with other things – like memory, sleep and sex life. It may also lead to symptoms like breathlessness and loss of appetite. The tiredness usually comes on during the first week or two of treatment, and often gets more apparent as the course of treatment continues. Once the chemotherapy is over, the sense of fatigue slowly reduces, but it can take anywhere from a month or two to more than a year before it completely disappears. Studies suggest that even a year after treatment has finished, about one in five people will still regularly have days when they feel fatigued. Generally speaking, the older the patient, the longer it takes to recover their stamina. Tiredness is also more likely if someone

is having, or has recently had, other treatments, like surgery or radiotherapy.

Although it is something that affects the majority of people, doctors have been slow to realize how important this tiredness is and have concentrated on more obvious side effects like sickness and the risk of infection. This means there has been relatively little research into the causes and treatment of chemotherapy-related fatigue. Chemotherapy itself undoubtedly does cause fatigue, but frequently there can be other factors that might make the feeling worse. These include anaemia, the presence of an infection, being clinically depressed or being in pain. All these are things that can often readily be corrected. So if someone does complain of feeling very tired, then it is important to make sure none of these other factors are present.

Anaemia can usually be rapidly reversed by a simple blood transfusion, which can often be given as an out-patient, or the use of erythropoeitic drugs. Even very mild levels of anaemia, with an Hb of 11g/L or less, which would not normally be troublesome, can lead to severe tiredness in people who are having chemotherapy, and correcting this can make a big difference to how they feel. Similarly giving antibiotics, or antifungal drugs, for an infection, or analgesics to relieve pain or prescribing antidepressants for people who are clinically depressed can ease their feeling of tiredness quite dramatically.

An important thing to remember is to reassure people that tiredness is a very common feature of chemotherapy, and it does not mean that their cancer is coming back, or getting worse, nor does it mean that things are going wrong with their treatment.

Hair Loss

For many people, the idea of having chemotherapy means that you must lose your hair. Alopecia is a major problem with cytotoxic treatment but not with most other types of cancer chemotherapy. The risk of hair loss is linked directly to which cytotoxic drugs are given, with some hair loss almost inevitable; with others it is virtually unknown (Table 2.7).

When hair loss occurs, it usually develops at about 3–4 weeks after starting treatment. Frequently, once it starts, it can progress very rapidly, with almost complete hair loss within a day or two, but sometimes it may be more a case of gradual thinning of the hair over several months. Scalp hair is the most sensitive to the effects of chemotherapy, because it grows more rapidly than hair on other parts of the body. But sometimes the drugs will cause loss of eyebrows, eyelashes, under-arm hair, and pubic hair as

TABLE 2.7. Cyototoxics and hair loss

Drugs which carry a high risk of total alopecia, or cosmetically significant hair loss

Cyclophosphamide	Etoposide
Dactinomycin	Ifosfamide
Daunorubicin	Irinotecan
Docetaxel	Paclitaxel
Doxorubicin	Temozolamide
Epirubicin	Vindesine

Drugs which sometimes cause noticeable hair loss, or thinning of the hair

Amsacrine	Lomustine
Bleomycin	Melphalan
Busulfan	Pemetrexed
Cytarabine	Pentostatin
Fludarabine	Topotecan
Fluorouracil	Vinblastine
Gemcitabine	Vincristine
Hydroxyurea	Vinorelbine
Idarubicin	

Drugs which rarely or never cause hair loss

Capecitabine	Mitomycin
Carboplatin	Mitoxantrone
Carmustine	Oxaliplatin
Chlorambucil	Procarbazine
Cisplatin	Raltitrexed
Cladribine	Tegafur
Dacarbazine	Thiotepa
Mercaptopurine	Tioguanine
Methotrexate	Treosulfan

well. As well as warning patients about the risk of hair loss, it is vital to remember to reassure them that, however much hair is lost, it will always grow back again. Normally the hair begins to reappear a month or so after the end of chemotherapy and is back completely within 3–6 months (sometimes it even starts to grow while people are still having the drugs). Often, however, it comes back with a different colour and appearance – a grey or black, 'pepper and salt' colouring, with quite a thick texture, and a slightly curly or wavy look is very common.

If treatment does involve drugs that carry a high risk of alopecia, the one thing that can sometimes be done to try to prevent, or reduce, this is scalp cooling. There are various types of scalp cooling, but the general principle is to chill the scalp, usually

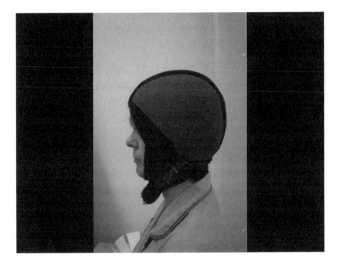

<small>Photo</small> 2.4. A typical 'cold cap' used for scalp cooling to prevent hair loss following cytotoxic chemotherapy (courtesy of the author) (*See* Color plate 3)

by wearing a special padded hat that contains a gel (Photo 4). The hat is stored in a freezer and is then strapped firmly on the patient's head about half an hour before they are due to have their drugs. They then continue to wear the hat for about half an hour after the drugs have been given. The underlying principle is that by keeping the scalp very cold the blood vessels in the scalp contract, so the blood supply to the hair follicles is reduced and they will be less affected by the circulating cytotoxics. Scalp cooling does not always work. For many people it will prevent or greatly reduce the amount of hair loss, but for others it has very little effect. One group of patients in whom it is often ineffective are those who have disturbed liver function, due to liver secondaries or other causes, which delays metabolism of many cytotoxic drugs, and hence maintains their concentration in the blood after the scalp cooling is complete. Some people find scalp cooling uncomfortable. The hat is very cold and can often cause headaches, so it does not suit everyone.

For those people who do develop alopecia the most obvious way of coping is having a wig. Most chemotherapy departments have a specially trained member of staff who can discuss the available options with and arrange a wig that meets the individual's colour and style. Alternatives to wigs include

TABLE 2.8. Advice for patients to reduce their risk of alopecia

- Avoid using heated products like curling tongs or heated rollers
- Try to wash your hair less often. The fewer times you wash your hair the better (but obviously you will have to find your own balance between reducing the frequency of washes and what you feel comfortable with)
- Avoid shampoos and conditioners with lots of chemicals: try using a baby shampoo
- Avoid hair dyes and colourants, unless they are completely organic (plant-based), with no added chemicals
- Avoid perms
- If you have very long hair, then having it cut to a shorter style may help

headscarves and bandanas, which allow some people to turn their hair loss into a fashion statement!

Patients often ask if there is anything that they can do to reduce the risk of hair loss, and Table 2.8 gives some useful tips.

Suggestion for further reading
Hesketh PJ, Batchelor D, Golant M. Chemotherapy-induced alopecia: psychosocial impact and therapeutic approaches. Supp Care Cancer, 2004; 12: 543–549.

Oral Mucositis
Having a sore mouth during chemotherapy is quite common as a result of inflammation of the lining of the mouth. The chances of getting a sore mouth do vary depending on the treatment;

TABLE 2.9. Cytotoxic drugs which commonly cause oral mucositis

Capecitabine	Hydroxyurea
Carboplatin	Lomustine
Chlorambucil	Melphalan
Cisplatin	Mercaptopurine
Cyclophosphamide	Methotrexate
Dacarbazine	Mitomycin
Dactinomycin,	Paclitaxel
Daunorubicin	Raltitrexed
Doxorubicin	Vinblastine
Etoposide	Vincristine
Fluorouracil	

some drugs, or combinations of drugs, are more likely to cause mucositis than others (Table 2.9). This oral mucositis usually comes on a few days after the drugs have been given and settles within about a week. The soreness can vary considerably in its severity. Often it is no more than a slight discomfort, but sometimes it can be very distressing, with the development of mucosal ulceration. Because the patient is often neutropenic as well, the soreness may be aggravated by the development of fungal infections in the mouth, most commonly oral monilia, which shows up as small whitish patches on the mucosa and the surface of the tongue. These infections are also common in people who are having steroids as part of their treatment. When mouth soreness develops it can also affect the sense of taste, so people often complain that things taste different, or that they cannot taste things so well whilst they are having their chemotherapy.

If a particular regimen is likely to cause mucositis then sucking crushed ice for 15–30 minutes before the cytotoxics are given, and continuing until about half an hour after the drugs have been administered, can sometimes prevent mouth soreness. One drug that is particularly associated with oral mucositis is methotrexate. The risk is usually dose-dependent and if higher doses of the drug are being used then giving an iv dose of folinic acid (leucovorin) at the same time as the methorexate and following this with a course of leucovorin tablets for a day or two can often prevent the problem (see P. 22). If mucositis does develop after methorexate administration, and folinic acid has not been given, then giving the tablets for a few days will often help. If patient does complain of a sore mouth after their chemotherapy then it is always important to check for the presence of oral monilia as this can readily be resolved with a course of an antifungal drug like nystatin, or amphotericin, for a few days. Oral soreness can also be eased by using a painkilling mouthwash such as Difflam Oral. Some people find using a full strength mouthwash stings, so diluting it with an equal amount of warm water may help. An alternative is to suggest patients make their own mouthwash using soluble aspirin, dissolving a couple of tablets in a glass of warm water and using this to rinse their mouth well three or four times a day. If mouth ulcers develop, then there is a wide range of gels, pastes and sprays that may help: these include Bonjela gel, Biora gel, Medijel and Rinstead contact pastilles.

More general advice for avoiding or easing oral mucositis includes ensuring that patients maintain good oral hygiene (Table 2.10) and changing their diet to avoid foods and drinks

TABLE 2.10. Advice for patients to reduce their risk of oral soreness

- Have a routine check-up with your dentist before you start treatment, to make sure there are no obvious tooth or gum problems that need to be dealt with before your chemotherapy.
- Maintain good oral hygiene; this means cleaning your teeth at least twice a day. Using a normal toothbrush can be uncomfortable, so using a soft toothbrush, or a child's brush, might help.
- You may find that your usual toothpaste makes your mouth and gums sore, and changing to a brand for 'sensitive teeth', like Sensodyne Original or Macleans Sensitive, might help.
- Mouthwashes can also be useful, and you can try these if you find that brushing your teeth is really painful. There are preparations you can get from your chemist or supermarket that help to prevent infection, these include chlorhexidine, Corsodyl and thymol.
- For simply keeping your mouth clean you can make your own mouthwash with a teaspoonful of baking powder (sodium bicarbonate) dissolved in a glass of warm water, and use this to rinse out your mouth thoroughly morning and night.
- Keeping your mouth moist with regular fluids. You should be drinking at least 2 litres of fluid every day during your treatment, but supplementing this with regular sips of water or other soft drinks can help (fizzy water, or fizzy drinks, tend to be better than still fluids)
- Try to avoid, or reduce, smoking, alcohol and caffeine (in tea and coffee) all of which tend to make your mouth dry and can make soreness worse

that may make their mouth sore if the mucosa is sensitive: these include very hot and spicy foods, vinegar, salt, neat spirits (whisky, brandy, gin, etc.) and acid drinks like grapefruit juice and some types of orange juice.

Suggestions for further reading

Keefe DM, Schubert MM, Elting LS et al. Updated clinical practice guidelines for the prevention and treatment of mucositis. Cancer, 2007; 109: 820–831.

Mitchell EP. Gastrointestinal toxicity of antineoplastic agents. Semin Oncol, 2006; 33: 106–120.

Reduced Fertility

As with other side effects, the risk of any effect on fertility is related to which drugs are used, and the doses given, and the duration of the treatment. Some cytotoxic treatments carry a very high risk of infertility, whereas with others there is almost no risk. The drugs that are most frequently associated with infertility are the alkylating agents. So if fertility is an issue then choosing regimens that either avoid these drugs completely, or keep their doses to a minimum, whilst maintaining anti-cancer efficacy, should be the objective. For example, in Hodgkin's disease (see P. 115), where young people are frequently affected, the original MOPP regimen, containing the potent alkylating agent nitrogen mustard leading to almost universal sterility, has largely been supplanted by ABVD, where the risk of infertility appears to be minimal.

For men, cytotoxics can have a direct effect on spermatogenesis, with a reduction in the sperm count becoming apparent within 3 weeks of starting the treatment. This risk relates almost entirely to which drugs are used (Table 2.11). But in some types of cancer, in particular cancer of the testicle, a reduced level of fertility, with a lower than normal sperm count, may actually be part of the man's condition, even before he begins any treatment.

TABLE 2.11. Chemotherapy and male fertility

Drugs likely to cause permanent or prolonged azoospermia

Busulfan	Ifosfamide
Carmustine	Lomustine
Chlorambucil	Melphalan
Cisplatin	Nitrogen mustard
Cyclophosphamide	Procarbazine
Dactinomycin	

Drugs which may cause some temporary reduction in sperm count when used alone, but can have an additive effect on fertility in combination regimens

Amsacrine	Fluorouracil
Bleomycin	Fludarabine
Carboplatin	Mercaptopurine
Cytaribine	Methotrexate
Dacarbazine	Mitoxantrone
Daunorubicin	Thioguanine
Doxorubicin	Thiotepa
Epirubicin	Vinblastine
Etoposide	Vincristine

Drugs with an unknown effect on spermatogenesis

Docetaxel	Oxaliplatin
Irinotecan	Paclitaxel
Monoclonal antibodies	Small molecule TK inhibitors

For women, cytotoxics may cause destruction of the ovarian follicles, resulting in failure of ovulation, amenorrhoea, and sterility. The drugs may also lead to a reduction in ovarian hormone production, leading to menopausal symptoms. The risk of loss of ovarian activity with cytotoxic treatment increases the closer a woman is to the natural menopause. Sometimes, especially in younger women, cytotoxic treatment leads only to a temporary loss of ovarian activity, so the periods stop during treatment, and for anywhere from 3 to 18 months afterwards, but can then start again. The risk of permanent ovarian suppression is confined to the alkylating agents and is largely dose dependent. Other drugs may cause a temporary interruption in ovarian function.

For men, if there is a chance that treatment will affect their fertility, they should always be offered the chance of sperm banking before beginning therapy. Freezing the sample does further reduce the quality of the sperm, but once they are frozen they can be kept indefinitely without any further deterioration and this does offer some hope of fathering future children. For women, the options are more limited. Freezing and storing of embryos that can be thawed and reimplanted into the womb after treatment is possible, but delaying treatment long enough for this to be arranged will not usually be possible. Even with this technique the chances of a successful pregnancy are probably still only about one in five. Taking away eggs (oocytes) from the ovary and having them frozen and taking away pieces of ovarian tissue for storage (that could be replaced after treatment to try and make the ovaries work again) are both possible, but are really experimental approaches that are still being developed with, at the moment, very little chance of success. Another option is egg donation where, after the treatment is over, the patient's womb could be implanted with eggs donated by another woman. This has resulted in successful pregnancies for some women after their ovaries have failed as a result of chemotherapy.

There are two other points to mention. Firstly, because of the unpredictability of the effects of cytotoxics on fertility, it would be wrong to think that having treatment acts as a reliable form of contraception. So if patients are practising birth control, they should be advised to continue it while they have their chemotherapy.

Secondly, people can be reassured that studies have shown that if fertility is reduced, but returns after chemotherapy, or if it was unaffected by treatment, the drugs that they have had will not lead to any increase in the chances of birth defects in children that they may father, or give birth to, in the future.

Suggestion for further reading

Lee SJ, Schover LR, Pertridge AH et al. American Society of Clinical Oncology recommendations on fertility preservation in cancer patients. J Clin Oncol, 2006; 24: 2917–2931.

Second Cancers

A number of cytotoxic drugs have been linked to the development of second malignancies, most commonly leading to acute myeloid leukaemia (AML). This problem was first identified following treatment with alkylating agents, in particular the nitrogen mustards. The risk varies with different agents (melphalan being some 10 times more potent a carcinogen than cyclophosphamide) and increases with the overall dose of the drug given. Typically the leukaemia appears some 5–9 years after treatment and is proceeded by the development of a myelodysplastic syndrome. Early estimates suggested that the likelihood of developing AML after alkylating agent therapy was about 1.5% at 10 years, but with greater awareness of the hazard this figure has probably reduced now.

The assumption is that it is the direct effect of alkylating agents on DNA that leads to their leukaemic potential and so other cytotoxics which interact directly with the DNA chain might be expected to pose similar risks. An increased incidence of AML has been identified following therapy with platinum compounds and the topoisomerase inhibitors (etoposide and the anthracyclines: epirubicin, doxorubicin and mitoxantrone). Isolated cases have also been reported after taxane-based chemotherapy. Among these drugs the risk appears to be highest with mitoxantrone with up to 4% of patients being affected, with the others there is less than a 1% chance of AML developing. Once again the risk appears to be related to dose-intensity, but unlike the AML linked to alkylating agents the onset is earlier, at 2–4 years post-treatment and not associated with an initial myelodysplastic phase.

Suggestions for further reading

Le Deley M-C, Suzan F, Cutuli B et al. Anthracyclines, mitoxantrone, radiotherapy, and granulocyte colony-stimulating factor: risk factors for leukemia and myelodysplastic syndrome after breast cancer. J Clin Oncol, 2007; 25: 292–300.

Praga C, Jonas B, Bliss J et al. Risk of acute myeloid leukemia and myelodysplastic syndrome in trials of adjuvant epirubicin for early breast cancer: correlation with doses of epirubicin and cyclophosphamide. J Clin Oncol, 2005; 23: 4179–4191.

Travis LB. The epidemiology of second primary cancers. Cancer Epidemiol & Biomarkers, 2006; 15: 2020–2026.

Specific Side Effects of Cytotoxic Treatment
There are a number of side effects of chemotherapy which, although important, and occasionally serious, are limited to just a handful of the more commonly used cytotoxic drugs.

Peripheral Neuropathy
The peripheral neuropathy caused by cytotoxic drugs is mainly sensory. The first symptom is tingling, or pins and needles, in the fingers or toes. This gradually spreads to the rest of the hands and feet and, if nothing is done, will go on to affect the rest of the limbs. As the condition progresses, numbness of the affected areas will develop, and this leads to some loss of co-ordination, making fine movements like undoing buttons, typing or tying shoelaces more difficult. Loss of reflexes in the ankle and wrist are relatively early physical signs but weakness of the arms and legs is a very uncommon, late, occurrence.

Peripheral neuropathy is a recognized complication of treatment with three groups of chemotherapy drugs: the Vinca alkaloids (which include vincristine, vinblastine, vindesine and vinorelbine), the platinum compounds (cisplatin, carboplatin and oxaliplatin) and the taxanes (paclitaxel and docetaxel). Of the Vinca alkaloids vincristine is the drug most likely to cause neuropathy, and it may also affect the autonomic nervous system leading to constipation and, very occasionally, intestinal obstruction. As well as causing a typical peripheral neuropathy, oxaliplatin is also linked to a specific syndrome where intense, often painful, tingling sensations occur in the fingers and toes a few hours after the drug is given, lasting from a few hours to a few days, the symptoms often being made worse by exposure to cold: up to 90% of people receiving oxaliplatin experience this problem.

Usually the peripheral neuropathy is dose related, and comes on gradually after two or three doses of the drugs, sometimes appearing only after treatment is complete. Numerous drugs have been used to try and prevent the neurotoxicity developing, but the results have been mixed and no one agent has been sufficiently successful to enter routine practice. If early signs of neuropathy appear then reducing the dose of the offending drug or stopping it completely will usually help ease the problem, but sometimes this is an unacceptable compromise of the treatment. The neuropathy resulting from both Vinca alkaloids and taxanes is generally reversible, although it may take months after treatment is over to disappear completely. With platinum compounds the picture is more mixed with the changes sometimes being permanent, although usually with low to moderate doses of the drugs there will be a recovery eventually.

Suggestions for further reading

Hausher FH, Schilsky RL, Berghonr EJ, Liberman F. Diagnosis, management and evaluation of chemotherapy-induced peripheral neuropathy. Semin Oncol, 2006; 33: 15–49.

Ocean AJ, Vahdat LT. Chemotherapy-induced peripheral neuropathy: pathogenesis and emerging treatments. Supp Care Cancer, 2004; 12: 619–625.

Cardiotoxicity

A number of cytotoxics carry the risk of cardiac damage, including the anthracyclines, fluorouracil and vinca alkaloids. Cardiotoxicity is also a side effect of the monoclonal antibody trastuzumab (see p. 74).

Doxorubicin is the anthracycline most likely to cause cardiac toxicity. Transient arrhythmias may occur in the first few hours after administration of the drug. These are most likely in people with previously abnormal ECGs. The arrhythmias usually do not require treatment and are not a contraindication to further doses of the drug. Very rarely more serious, life-threatening, ventricular arrhythmias have been reported. The more significant risk with the drug is chronic cardiomyopathy. This is dose-related. Early studies suggested that less than 1% of people who received a cumulative dose of <550mg/m²were affected, with the incidence increasing to more than 30% with cumulative doses between 550 and 1150mg/m². With greater awareness of this problem, and better means of monitoring it, particularly the measurement of left ventricular ejection fraction (LVEF), it is now clear that the incidence may be higher and cardiac damage can occur even at relatively low doses. For these reasons many clinicians have reduced the maximum cumulative dose of the drug to 450–500mg/m². The cardiomyopathy leads to congestive cardiac failure, which may not appear until some months, or even years, after the last dose of the drug. The heart failure can often be difficult to treat and carries quite a high mortality. Apart from dose, other predisposing factors include age over 70, pre-existing heart disease and a past history of radiotherapy to the mediastinum. Most dose schedules for doxorubicin give total doses below the 500mg/m² level. For those people with risk factors that might lead to problems at lower levels, monitoring of their LVEF is advisable; a pre-treatment value of 45% or a fall to this level during treatment would usually indicate that the drug is contra-indicated or should be stopped. Epirubicin has the potential to cause similar cardiac problems to doxorubicin, but the cumulative dose at which these are seen is significantly higher, at between 900 and 1000mg/m^2. Chronic cardiomyopathy may occur with other anthracyclines, and once again is dose related: with daunorubicin at a cumulative dose below 500mg/m^2 1.5% of people will develop cardiomyopathy, whereas between 500 and 100mg/m^2 the figure rises to 12% and for mitoxantrone the suggested maximum cumulative dose is 160mg/m^2.

A number of suggestions have been made to reduce doxorubicin toxicity. There is limited evidence that the risk of cardiac damage is reduced if the drug is given by prolonged intravenous infusion, or on a weekly basis at lower doses. Also a number of agents have been investigated as cardioprotective agents during doxorubicin therapy, the most widely evaluated being dexrazoxane, but their value remains to be established. The liposomal formulation of doxorubicin does not permeate the blood vessels of the myocardium and is associated with only minimal cardiotoxicity.

A further problem with doxorubicin is that when given in combination with paclitaxel there is a high risk of cardiotoxicity. Studies have now shown that this relates to the scheduling of the drugs, as the paclitaxel infusion delays doxorubicin clearance and prolongs its plasma half-life. The risk of cardiac damage can be minimized by giving doxorubicin first, with a delay of at least 30 minutes before the paclitaxel infusion, and limiting the cumulative dose of doxorubicin during treatment to 360mg/m^2. By contrast, combining doxorubicin with docetaxel is not associated with an increased risk of cardiac damage, nor is there any increased risk if either taxane is given with epirubicin.

Both fluorouracil and capecitabine may cause cardiotoxicity. The signs of this range from asymptomatic ECG changes to angina pectoris and myocardial infarction, which may be fatal. The mechanism for these changes remains uncertain, although coronary vasospasm has been suggested. With fluorouracil they are most likely to occur within 72 hours of the first dose of the drug and are common with higher doses given by continuous infusion. When symptoms occur about half the patients experience angina, about 25% infarction, 15% arrhythmias and the remainder either acute pulmonary oedema, pericarditis or cardiac arrest. The development of cardiotoxicity means that the drug should be stopped, and in trials where patients have been rechallenged with fluorouracil after signs of cardiac problems, there have been significant numbers of cardiac deaths.

Suggestions for further reading

Ng R, Better N, Green MD. Anti-cancer agents and cardiotoxicity. Semin Oncol, 2006; 33: 2–14.

Renal Damage

Cisplatin is the cytotoxic drug most closely associated with nephrotoxicity. The degree of injury to the kidneys is dose-dependent, and cumulative, single doses below 50mg/m^2 seldom cause problems. Higher doses lead to renal tubular injury which in turn may lead to electrolyte imbalance, especially low sodium and/or magnesium levels in the blood, as well as reduced creatinine clearance levels and ultimately renal failure. These changes persist for months, and often years, after treatment is over; for example, it has been estimated that 4 years after chemotherapy with cisplatin men treated for testicular cancer have, on average, a 15% reduction in their creatinine clearance.

As well as dose-limitation cisplatin nephrotoxicity can also be reduced by using a forced diuresis, with large volumes of intravenous normal saline before and after administration of the drug. This dilutes the concentration of cisplatin in the renal tubules and speeds its transit through the kidneys. Originally the schedules for the saline infusions lasted anywhere from 24 to 36 hours, necessitating that treatment be given on an in-patient basis, but these have been modified over time and it is now often possible to give the treatment on a day-patient basis. A number of chemicals have been evaluated as possible agents to reduce the renal toxicity of cisplatin, the most widely tested being amifostine, but none of these has proved sufficiently successful to enter routine practice.

Carboplatin was developed as an analogue of cisplatin specifically to find a less nephrotoxic alternative. Carboplatin does cause less damage to the kidneys, only causing problems when given at high doses, but it does carry a greater risk of myelosuppression than cisplatin. To minimize the risk of renal damage carboplatin dosing is directly related to renal function (see page 35).

Other cytotoxics that have been linked to renal damage include mitomycin, methotrexate and ifosfamide. Problems usually occur only with either prolonged cumulative administration or higher than normal individual doses.

Suggestion for further reading

deJonge MJA, Verweij J. Renal toxicities of chemotherapy. Semin Oncol, 2006; 33: 68–73.

Hepatotoxicity

Three types of liver damage have been linked to cytotoxic drugs: hepatocellular dysfunction, veno-occlusive disease and chronic fibrosis.

Hepatocellular dysfunction is characterized by an increase in the blood level of liver enzymes and bilirubin. It has most often been reported with high-dose cytarabine therapy and mercaptopurine but it may occur occasionally as a result of a number of other drugs (Table 2.12).

Veno-occlusive disease leads to blockage of small blood vessels in the liver which in turn causes hepatomegaly, ascites and oedema, and may progress to be fatal. It has been reported after high-dose therapy with a number of alkylating agents and also in isolated instances with a number of other cytotoxics.

Hepatic fibrosis is a complication of long-term low-dose methotrexate administration. The drug is usually only given in this way in the treatment of a number of non-malignant conditions, such as rheumatoid arthritis.

Suggestion for further reading

Floyd J, Mirza I, Sachs B, Perry MC. Hepatotoxicity of chemotherapy. Semin Oncol, 2006; 33: 50–67.

TABLE 2.12. Cytotoxic hepatotoxicity

Hepatotoxicity	Recognised side effect	Isolated reports
Hepatocellular toxicity	cytarabine* mercaptopurine	chlorambucil gemcitabine raltitrexed
Veno-occlusive disease	busulfan* carmustine* cyclophosphamide cytarabine mitomycin	dacarbazine gemcitabine mercaptopurine thioguanine
Chronic fibrosis	methotrexate	

* Following high-dose therapy.

Pulmonary Toxicity

Bleomycin is the cytotoxic most widely associated with lung damage, leading to chronic pulmonary fibrosis. Some estimates suggest as many as 1 in 10 people receiving the drug may be affected. Typically the changes appear 1–6 months after treatment. The pulmonary toxicity is dose related and usually only appears when more than 400,000–500,000 units of the drug have been given (bleomycin dose-labelling varies in different parts of the world, and outside Europe this equates to 400–500 units). Other factors predisposing to drug-induced pulmonary fibrosis include older age, poor renal function (delaying excretion of the drug, allowing it to concentrate in the lungs) and radiotherapy to the chest. Much less commonly, bleomycin may cause an early onset interstitial pneumonitis, which may also lead to long-term fibrosis in some cases; this is not dose related and is similar to a hypersensitivity reaction.

Mitomycin can cause a range of pulmonary toxicities ranging from transient bronchospasm, which resolves spontaneously a few hours after the drug has been given, to acute interstitial pneumonitis, chronic pneumonitis and pulmonary fibrosis. Other drugs where lung toxicity, predominantly pulmonary fibrosis, has occasionally been reported include busulfan (the first cytotoxic to be linked to lung damage), methotrexate, cyclophosphamide, the taxanes and the vinca alkaloids.

Suggestion for further reading

Meadors M, Floyd J, Perry MC. Pulmonary toxicity of chemotherapy. Semin Oncol 2006; 33: 98–105.

Skin Damage

Cytotoxic drugs may affect the skin in a number of ways but the two most important are extravasation (leakage of the drug outside the vein at the injection site) and hand–foot syndrome.

When cytotoxic drugs are given through a drip into a peripheral vein, even when the drug is given carefully, by trained skilled nurses, small amounts of the drug may occasionally leak outside the vein, into the surrounding soft tissues. It has been estimated that some degree of extravasation may occur in up to 5% of patients undergoing intravenous chemotherapy. With many drugs, extravasation is not a problem and, at most, will only cause some slight brief discomfort. With a few drugs, however, any leakage into the tissues around the vein can cause quite severe inflammation, with redness, swelling and soreness (Photo 5). This comes on almost immediately after the extravasation has occurred and, depending on the drug and the amount that has

Anthracycline extravasation –
day 4 redness & swelling

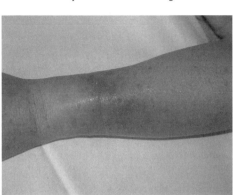

PHOTO 2.5. Skin reaction 4 days after anthracycline extravasation: redness, swelling and induration (courtesy of Mr David Bobs, Topo Target A/S) (*See* Color plate 4)

leaked into the tissues it may take days, or even weeks, to resolve. Occasionally long-term induration or even skin necrosis can result (Photo 6). The drugs most likely to cause irritation and skin damage when they leak are the anthracyclines, doxorubicin and epirubicin, the Vinca alkaloids, vincristine, vinblastine, vindesine and vinorelbine and the taxane, paclitaxel.

If extravasation occurs then the tube through which the drug is being infused should be disconnected, but the needle into the vein should remain in place. A syringe can then be connected to the needle and used to draw back any remaining drug. Ice packs should then be placed on the surrounding skin, and the arm kept elevated. In addition specific antidotes have been recommended. For anthracycline extravasation topical application of dimethyl sulfoxide may help and more recently intravenous infusions of dexrasoxane, started within 6 hours of the leakage, have also been shown to be of value. For Vinca alkaloid and paclitaxel leakage immediate local subcutaneous injection of hyaluronidase is beneficial. Using an anti-inflammatory or antihistamine cream on the affected area for a week or so afterwards can also help. Very occasionally if chronic painful skin damage results hyperbaric oxygen therapy, or surgery, with removal of the affected soft tissues and skin grafting may be necessary.

In recent years cytotoxic extravasation has featured increasingly in legal claims by patients. So if it does occur then it

Anthracycline extravasation –
day 12 necrosis

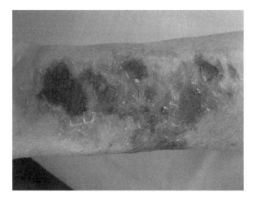

PHOTO 2.6. Skin reaction 12 days after severe anthracycline extravasation: blistering and necrosis. This picture and Photo 2.5 one show typical skin reactions prior to the availability of dexrazoxane (Savene™) as a treatment for it (courtesy of Mr David Bobs, Topo Target A/S) (*See* Color plate 5)

should not only be treated meticulously, but also all aspects of the incident should be carefully documented.

A completely different type of skin damage which can occur with a number of cytotoxic drugs including fluorouracil, capecitabine, irinotecan, the taxanes and cytarabine is hand–foot syndrome (also known as palmar-plantar erythrodysesthesia, or acral erythema). In hand–foot syndrome the skin on the palms of the hands and soles of the feet becomes red and sore and may actually begin to blister and peel. Sometimes the pain from this can be so severe that narcotic analgesics are needed to control it. It usually only comes on gradually with higher does of the drugs, and adjusting the dose will often ease the problem. Sometimes taking tablets of Vitamin B6 (pyridoxine) at a dose of 200mg daily will give some symptomatic relief.

Suggestions for further reading

Goolsby TV, Lombardo FA. Extravasation of chemotherapeutic agents: prevention and treatment. Semin Oncol 2006; 33: 139–143.

Mouridsen HT, Langer SW, Buter J et al. Treatment of anthracycline extravasation with Savene (desrasoxane): results from two prospective multicentre studies. Annals Oncol, 2007; 18: 546–550.

Shahab N, Haider S, Doll DC. Vascular toxicity of antineoplastic agents. Semin Oncol 2006; 33: 121–138.

Ototoxicity

Cisplatin damages the outer hair cells in the organ of Corti in the inner ear. This injury can lead to symptoms ranging from reversible tinnitus to irreversible hearing loss and vestibular toxicity. The risk of ototoxicity is dose and schedule dependent, being uncommon with doses of $<60mg/m^2$ per cycle. A number of drugs have been tried as agents to protect against cisplatin-induced ototoxicity, but none has so far proved successful. As a result dose reduction is the only way of preventing severe, irreversible hearing loss.

Suggestion for further reading

Rademaker-Lakhai JM, Crul M, Zuur L et al. Relationship between cisplatin administration and the development of ototoxicity. J Clin Oncol, 2006; 24: 918–924.

Bladder Toxicity

The alkylating agents, ifosfamide and cyclophosphamide, when metabolized produce a number of chemicals which are excreted in the urine. A number of these are urotoxic and can cause irritation to the urothelium, leading to haemorrhagic cystitis. This is usually only a problem with cyclophosphamide when the drug is given at high doses, but with ifosfamide it is a risk at standard doses of the drug. The main urotoxic chemical which is produced is acrolein and this can be neutralized by mercaptoethanesulfonate (MESNA). MESNA is routinely given as an iv infusion at the same time as ifosfamide, and it binds with acrolein, and other metabolites, to form stable non-urotoxic compounds which are rapidly excreted. MESNA does not have any anti-cancer action in its own right, nor does it reduce the effectiveness of the ifasfamide.

Diarrhoea and Constipation

Diarrheoa is most likely to occur following the administration of either fluorouracil, capecitabine or irinotecan. Depending on the dose and schedule used, this can be severe, or even life-threatening, and patients should always be made aware of this risk. For mild to moderate diarrheoa (the passage of stool 4–6 times daily) dietary advice combined with regular doses of loperamide and a good fluid intake to avoid dehydration should suffice. If the mild to moderate diarrheoa is accompanied by any complicating factors (Table 2.13), or if the diarrheoa is more severe, with the passage of stool seven or more times daily, then more aggressive management is indicated. This would normally involve admitting the patient for intravenous hydration,

TABLE 2.13. Factors complicating diarrhoea

Severe abdominal cramping
Grade II or greater nausea or vomiting
Reduced performance status
Fever
Sepsis
Neutropenia
Obvious rectal bleeding
Dehydration

and subcutaneous or intravenous injections of the somatostatin analogue, octreotide, titrating the dose as necessary to bring the situation under control.

Constipation is most commonly seen with vincristine therapy, and usually appears 3–4 days after the drug is given. It is due to the effects of vincristine on the autonomic nerves and may often be accompanied by signs of peripheral neuropathy. It is more likely in elderly patients or those on higher doses of the drug. Usually it will respond to mild laxatives and stool softeners, but occasionally it can progress to a paralytic ileus. This will usually resolve with conservative management over 7–10 days.

Suggestions for further reading
Benson AB, Jaffer AA, Catalano RB et al. J Clin Oncol, 2004; 22: 2918–2926.
Gibson RJ, Keefe DMK. Cancer chemotherapy-induced diarrhea and constipation: mechanisms of damage and prevention strategies. Supp Care Cancer, 2006; 14: 890–900.

Hypersensitivity Reactions
These are most likely to be seen with the taxanes (Table 2.14). The reaction is apparent within moments of starting the infusion and may include blood pressure changes (hypotension or hypertension), breathlessness, severe anxiety, flushing, a diffuse erythema, angioedema, itching and chest pain. The reaction is caused by sensitivity to solutes necessary to get the active drugs into solution (Cremophor for paclitaxel, Tween 80 for docetaxel) rather than by the drugs themselves. The risk of reactions can be reduced by premedication. For paclitaxel this involves giving the steroid dexamethasone, together with an antihistamine and an H2 antagonist, for docetaxel usually only dexamethasone is given. Giving dexamethasone prior to docetaxel administration also reduces the risk of another complication of the drug: fluid retention, which can lead to oedema, pleural or pericardial

TABLE 2.14. Cytotoxic drugs likely to cause hypersensitivity reactions

Drug	Incidence of reactions
Bleomycin	1%
Carboplatin	5%
Docetaxel	20% (4% severe)
Doxorubicin (liposomal)	10%
Etoposide iv	2%
Oxaliplatin	20% (3% severe)
Paclitaxel	40% (2% severe)

effusions or ascites. If a reaction does occur then the infusion should be stopped immediately and changed to intravenous saline, intravenous hydrocortisone and antihistamine should be given, and oxygen administered. In severe cases adrenalin may be necessary. The symptoms will usually rapidly subside, and often the infusion can be restarted after 30 minutes without further problems.

Liposomal doxorubicin causes similar immediate reactions in about 10% of patients, although the episodes are usually less severe. They occur only with first infusions. For those patients who give a history of allergies, premedication with a steroid and an antihistamine may be a wise precaution.

In contrast to the taxane hypersensitivity reactions, those seen with oxaliplatin and carboplatin tend to occur only after a number of courses of the drug have been given, typically 6–8 cycles. A number of desensitization protocols have been reported which may prevent further reactions, but often the development of hypersensitivity necessitates stopping the drug completely.

Acute hypersensitivity reactions have been reported with many other cytotoxics but they occur only rarely.

Suggestions for further reading
de Lemos M. Acute reactions to chemotherapy agents. J Oncol Pharm Pract, 2006; 12: 127–129.
Markman M. Managing taxane toxicities. Supp Care Cancer, 2003; 11: 144–147.
Weiss RB. Miscellaneous toxicities. In DeVita VT, Hellman S, Rossenberg SA. Cancer: principles and practice of oncology, 7th edition. Lippincott, Williams & Wilkins, 2005, 2602–2614.

Tumour Lysis Syndrome
This is usually only seen with bulky, highly chemosensitive tumours, or in leukaemias with high blast counts. When

cytotoxics are first given in the treatment of these cancers they may cause massive tumour necrosis which can lead to acute biochemical disturbances including hyperuricaemia, hyperkalaemia, hyperphosphataemia and hypocalcaemia. These can lead to acidosis and acute renal failure. Patients whose serum uric acid level or lactic dehydrogenase level (LDH) is raised prior to treatment, or those with poor renal function, are particularly at risk. The key to management of this complication is prevention. Patients who are deemed to be at risk would usually be given oral allopurinol, to reduce their uric acid levels, prior to starting chemotherapy, and continue this throughout their treatment. This, combined with ensuring a good fluid intake, will usually be sufficient prophylaxis. If the syndrome does develop then giving allopurinol, if it has not already been given, intravenous hydration and urinary alkalinization are the first line management. If allopurinol has already been given then rasburicase may be used as an alternative. This is a recombinant form of the enzyme urate oxidase, which converts poorly soluble uric acid to water-soluble metabolites. In severe cases it may be necessary to consider renal dialysis.

SIDE EFFECTS OF HORMONAL TREATMENT

Menopausal Symptoms

Generally hormone therapies cause fewer, and less serious, side effects than chemotherapy. Many women being treated for breast cancer have virtually no problems at all from their hormonal treatment. Having said this, for a small minority of women the therapy can be very upsetting. The most common problems are unpleasant menopausal side effects. These include hot-flushes, drenching sweats, vaginal dryness and soreness, mood swings, and irritability, loss of concentration and difficulty in remembering things. These are most likely to occur with tamoxifen, or goserelin. In younger women who are taking tamoxifen, about one-third will find their periods stop (if this happens it is still possible for the woman to become pregnant and she should continue contraception), one-third will find they become irregular, and one-third will see no difference, but all may get menopausal symptoms, as may some women who are postmenopausal and are given the drug. A variety of things can be done to try and ease these symptoms, and because this is a very common problem these will be described in more detail.

If the symptoms are due to tamoxifen then changing the way the drug is taken might make a difference: either altering

Color Plates

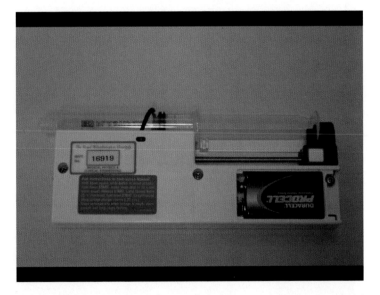

COLOR PLATE 1. A battery-driven chemotherapy pump (courtesy of Mr Simon Glazebrook, New Cross Hospital Wolverhampton)

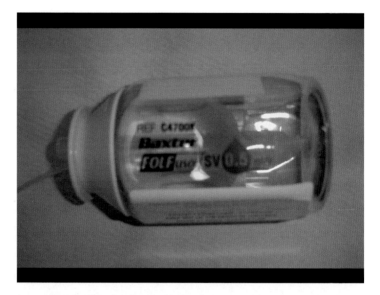

Color Plate 2. A disposable elastomeric infusion pump (courtesy of Mr Simon Glazebrook, New Cross Hospital Wolverhampton)

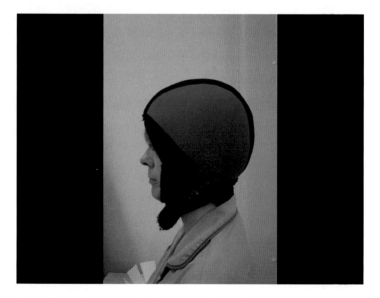

Color Plate 3. A typical 'cold cap' used for scalp cooling to prevent hair loss following cytotoic chemotherapy (courtesy of the author)

Anthracycline extravasation –
day 4 redness & swelling

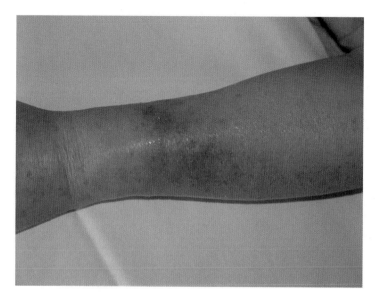

COLOR PLATE 4. Skin reaction 4 days after anthracycline extravasation:
redness, swelling and induration (courtesy of Mr David Bobs, Topo
Target A/S)

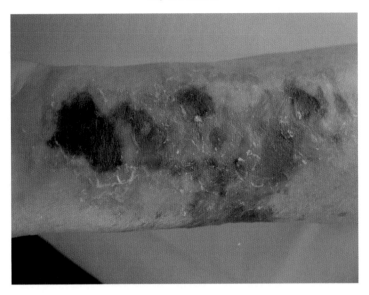

Color Plate 5. Skin reaction 12 days after severe anthracycline extravasation: blistering and necrosis. This picture and photograph 5 one show typical skin reactions prior to the availability of dexrazoxane (Savene™) as a treatment for it (courtesy of Mr David Bobs, Topo Target A/S)

the time of day that it is taken or breaking the tablet in two and taking half in the morning and half at night. Tamoxifen is made by a number of different manufacturers, and although all their products contain the same active drug, some women find that changing from one brand of tamoxifen to another does make a difference to their symptoms. If none of these help then, for women who are past their menopause, a change from tamoxifen to an aromatase inhibitor, like anastrazole, letrozole or exemestane, might well help and will not affect the efficacy of treatment.

Sometimes simple lifestyle changes make things easier. Regular exercise, losing weight, and avoiding certain foods, particularly spicy foods, and certain drinks, particularly alcohol, may help to reduce the problem. Complementary therapies may also make a difference. There are a number of preparations available from pharmacists and health food shops which contain plant oestrogens (phyto oestrogens), the active ingredients include red clover, soy, genistein and black cohosh. There has been anxiety that because these compounds are a form of oestrogen, they might increase the risk of breast cancer recurrence but there is no evidence that this is the case. Vitamin E supplements have also been shown to help in some studies. Evening primrose oil and ginseng are other popular remedies, and many women feel they reduce the number and severity of hot flushes and sweats, although scientific evidence for this is scarce. Studies have shown, however, that both acupuncture and relaxation therapies can benefit some women.

Sometimes prescription drugs may improve the situation. The options here include low doses of the female hormone progesterone, certain types of antidepressants and clonidine (which alters the blood vessel tone). None of these is a sure way of improving the problem, but if the symptoms are severe and troublesome they might be worth trying. The role of hormone replacement therapy (HRT) is controversial. Certainly it is often very effective at relieving the symptoms, but its safety is in question. At least one large clinical trial shows that women who use HRT after a diagnosis of breast cancer have an increased risk of recurrence, but this risk only seems to affect women over 50. So up to that age HRT may be given but thereafter, unless symptoms are very severe and all else has failed, HRT is not to be recommended. An alternative might be the drug tibilone, which has some oestrogen-like activity, and seems as effective as HRT in easing flushes and sweats. One study has suggested that it might lead to a slight increase in the risk of breast cancer coming back, but a large clinical trial is currently underway to determine exactly how useful, and how safe, it is.

Suggestions for further reading

Gainford M, Simmons C, Nguyen H et al. A practical guide to the management of menopausal symptoms in breast cancer patients. Supp Care Cancer, 2005; 13: 573–578.

Hickey M, Davis SR, Sturdee DW. Treatment of menopausal symptoms: what shall we do now? Lancet, 2005; 366: 409–421.

Nelson HD, Kimberly KV, Haney E et al. Non-hormonal therapies for menopausal hot flashes: systematic review and meta-analysis. J Am Med Assoc, 2006; 295: 2057–2071.

Endometrial Cancer

Long-term tamoxifen therapy is associated with a small but definite risk of developing cancer of the womb. Approximately 1 in 500 women taking tamoxifen for more than 2 years will develop endometrial cancer. This is because tamoxifen affects different oestrogen receptors differently, inhibiting those in breast cancer cells, but stimulating those in the endometrium, leading to endometrial hyperplasia, and ultimately endometrial cancer. For this reason post-menopausal women who are taking tamoxifen should always be warned to report any vaginal bleeding so that this can rapidly be investigated to exclude the possibility of cancer. Happily most endometrial cancers related to tamoxifen therapy have been detected at any early stage, and the cure rate has been high.

Thromboembolic Disease

Another consequence of the oestrogenic properties of tamoxifen is an increased risk of venous thrombosis. The risk is quite small with less than 1% of women taking tamoxifen getting deep vein thromboses. It is, however, advisable that women with a history of venous thrombosis should have an alternative therapy, such as an aromatase inhibitor, if possible.

Osteoporosis

The reduction in oestrogen level that occurs after the menopause means that older women are prone to develop osteoporosis. Use of aromatase inhibitors increases this risk. Exemestane is a steroidal aromatase inhibitor, in contrast to anastrazole and letrozole, and it has been suggested that it might be less likely to lead to a loss of bone mineral density. Whilst this is probably true, there is still an increased risk of osteoporosis even with this drug. Osteoporosis increases the risk of bone fractures, and these appear to be about 50% more common in women on an aromatase inhibitor than those on tamoxifen (the adverse effect of aromatase inhibitors on bone mineral density is in contrast to tamoxifen, which has a mild oestrogenic action on the bones, and hence offers some protection against osteoporosis). Although there are no definite national guidelines in the UK, it is generally recommended that women who are to receive aromatase inhibitors have a baseline bone densitometry, DXA scan, of their hip and lumbar spine prior to starting treatment. Depending on the result of this, they may simply need advice on lifestyle measures to reduce the risk of osteoporosis (such as stopping smoking, reducing alcohol consumption, taking regular exercise and eating a healthy diet), or be advised to take vitamin D and calcium supplements. For women at high risk then adding a bisphosphonate, such as alendronic acid or risedronate sodium, to their drug regimen may be indicated.

Hormonal Therapies for Prostate Cancer
The gonaderilin analogues, goserelin and leuprorelin, usually have relatively few side effects. The most important of these is the risk of tumour flare in metastatic disease, when the drugs may initially cause a surge in androgen production during the first 2 weeks of their administration, before inhibiting release of the male hormones. This can be avoided by giving an anti-androgen at the same time as the gonaderilin analogue. Other side effects which may occur include 'menopausal' hot flushes and sweats, loss of libido and impotence, and irreversible breast pain and swelling (gynaecomastia).

The anti-androgens may also lead to gynaecomastia, breast pain and 'menopausal' hot flushes. Giving a low dose of radiotherapy to the nipple area before starting the drugs can often prevent the development of gynaecomastia, similarly giving tamoxifen may also prevent breast swelling and pain. Because they do not reduce circulating androgen levels the non-steroidal anti-androgens, bicalutamide and flutamide, do not usually reduce libido or cause problems with erectile function or osteoporosis, whereas these may happen with the steroidal preparation, cyproterone. In addition cyproterone carries the risk of hepatotoxicity. The other main systemic hormonal therapy for prostate cancer, stilboestrol, carries the risk of cardiovascular toxicity due to thromboembolic complications.

Suggestions for further reading

Lester J, Dodwell D, McLoskey E, Coleman R. The causes and treatment of bone loss associated with cancer of the breast. Cancer Treat Rev, 2005; 31: 115–142.

Shapiro CL. Aromatase inhibitors and bone loss: the risks in perspective. J Clin Oncol, 2005; 23: 4847–4849.

SIDE EFFECTS OF TARGETED THERAPIES

By definition, targeted therapies specifically attack cancer cells, with little or no effect on normal tissues – in direct contrast to cytotoxic drugs, which have similar actions on normal and malignant cells. Consequently targeted therapies generally have fewer, and less severe, side effects than cytotoxic drugs. These are summarized in Table 2.15, but a few features do merit further explanation.

Trastuzumab and Cardiotoxicity

When used as a single agent trastuzumab causes symptomatic cardiac failure in up to 5% of patients. However, when it is given with either anthracycline cytotoxics or paclitaxel the rate of cardiac failure is much higher, reaching 25% in some studies, with a number of cases being severe. It has been suggested that this is because trastuzumab inhibits the mechanisms which repair myocardial damage caused by the cytotoxics. The resulting cardiac failure can be treated by standard therapies, and in the great majority of patients it is reversible once the drug is withdrawn.

Infusion Reactions: Cytokine Release Syndrome

Infusion reactions are common with the monoclonal antibodies and most often appear as hypersensitivity reactions with symptoms such as chills, fever, and an urticarial rash. Occasionally a more serious reaction may develop: cytokine release syndrome. This is thought to be due to monoclonal antibodies stimulating white blood cells to release large amounts of cytotokines which produce an acute systemic inflammatory reaction. The most prominent symptom is severe dyspnoea, often with bronchospasm. As with the hypersensitivity reactions, chills, rigors, urticaria and angioedema are also frequently present but in contrast to those reactions cytokine release syndrome usually appears 1–2 hours after the infusion has commenced, rather than in the first few minutes of an infusion. Cytokine release syndrome is also often accompanied by signs of tumour lysis syndrome

TABLE 2.15. Summary of side effects of targeted therapies

	Alemtuzumab	Bevacizumab	Bortezomib	Cetuximab	Dasatinib	Erlotinib	Gefitinib	Imatinib
Infusion reactions	+			+				
Fever/flu like symptoms			+					
Skin rash	+			+			+	
Cardiotoxicity								+
Hypertension		+				+		
Hypotension	+		+					
Haemorrhage								
Thrombosis		+						
Nausea			+			+		+
Diarrhoea	+		+			+		+
Constipation	+							
Fatigue			+			+		+
Alopecia								
Neuropathy			+					
Muscle/joint pain	+		+					+
Headache			+					+
Myelosuppression			+		+			
Oedema								+
Pleural effusion					+			
G-I perforation		+						

TABLE 2.15. (continued)

	Lapatinib	Nilotinib	Rituximab	Sorafinib	Sunitinib	Thalidomide	Trastuzumab
Infusion reactions			+				+
Fever/ flu-like symptoms			+			+	+
Skin rash	+	+		+			
Hand foot syndrome				+	+		
Pruritis	+			+			
Cardiotoxicity							+
Hypertension				+	+		
Hypotension			+				
Thrombosis						+	
Nausea	+		+	+			
Diarrhoea	+		+	+	+		+
Constipation				+		+	
Fatigue	+			+	+	+	
Sedation						+	
Cardiotoxicity				+			
Neuropathy						+	
Muscle/joint pain							+
Headache							+
Myelosuppression		+				+	+
Tumour pain			+				+
Raised biliribun		+				+	

(see P. 69), with hyperuricaemia and hypercalcaemia. Cytokine release syndrome is a potentially fatal complication of treatment and requires emergency treatment. It is most likely in patients with a high tumour burden and those with pre-existing lung disease. If possible, alternative treatments should be used for these patients. Cytokine release syndrome has most often been reported with rituximab and alemtuzumab but may rarely occur with other anti-cancer monoclonal antibodies.

Targeted Therapies and Skin Toxicity

About 80% of patients given cetuximab, and a majority receiving erlotinib and gefitinib, will develop an acneiform skin rash within the first week or two of treatment, for some this will be quite severe. Although labelled acneiform, the rash is not true acne and routine acne medications, such as benzoyl peroxide, should be avoided. It can appear as either a pustular eruption or a pustulo/papular or a follicular rash. There is no universally agreed treatment but routine measures include the use of mild soaps and skin moisturisers, with topical or systemic antibiotics if there is evidence of secondary infection (which is quite common). For more troublesome macular rashes topical steroids may help and for pusutular rashes topical clindamycin may be beneficial. The rash usually fades spontaneously after a few weeks, leaving the skin dry and liable to crack. An unusual feature of the rash is that people who suffer a more severe reaction are more likely to gain a therapeutic response.

Suggestions for further reading

Ng R, Better N, Green MD. Anti-cancer agents and cardiotoxicity. Semin Oncol, 2006; 33: 2–14.

Sipples R. Common side effects of anti-EGFR therapy: acneform rash. Semin Oncol Nursing, 2006; 22: 28–34.

Part 3
Chemotherapy in the Management of Cancer

BREAST CANCER

Breast cancer is now the commonest cancer in UK. Every year more than 40,000 women, and 300 men, will find they have breast cancer. Overall nearly one in nine women will develop the condition at some time during their lives. The risk of getting the disease increases with age: half of all breast cancers are first diagnosed in women over the age of 65, and a quarter are first diagnosed in women over the age of 75. Breast cancer is becoming more common. The number of new cases each year in the UK has almost doubled over the last 40 years. Although this increase in the frequency of the disease is worrying, it is offset by the fact that the cure rate is rapidly improving. In the early 1990s only about half of all women who had breast cancer could expect to live 10 years or more, but now this figure has increased to more than seven out of ten and is expected to improve further over the coming years.

Oncologists have debated whether this improvement is due to the introduction of breast screening, with the detection of cancers at an earlier, more curable, stage, or the introduction of adjuvant chemotherapy. Statisticians suggest that probably the latter is the major factor, contributing more than 60% to the increase in life-expectancy. When considering the use of adjuvant chemotherapy in early breast cancer two key questions are as follows: Who should receive treatment and what treatment should they receive? One way to answer these complex issues is to adopt an historical approach.

Following the publication of the results from the early adjuvant studies in the 1970s it was possible, by 1980, to make clear recommendations. In terms of patient selection those women who had axillary node involvement at the time of their initial surgery should be offered systemic adjuvant therapy, whereas this treatment was not necessary for those women whose cancers were node negative. When it came to choosing what drugs to use the evidence suggested that pre-menopausal women should receive cytotoxic drugs, most frequently with the classical combination of cyclophosphamide, methorexate and fluorouracil (CMF), and post-menopausal women should be given hormonal therapy, with tamoxifen.

Over the last 25 years it has become apparent that tumour size and the histological grade of the cancer are important prognostic factors, as well as the axillary node status. As a consequence selection criteria have been adjusted to allow for these additional variables. But there is no absolute consensus as to how these criteria should be applied to individual patients. Currently at least three systems are available to make this decision. These are personal experience, prognostic formulae and 'Adjuvant on line'. Personal experience relies on the judgement of individual specialists or groups of experts in multidisciplinary teams making decisions based on their knowledge and skill. The prognostic formulae take the patient's details, put them into an equation and produce a number indicating their risk of recurrent disease. The most widely used of these calculations is the Nottingham Prognostic Index, which is as follows:

Tumour size (cm × 0.2) + lymph node stage (1 = node negative, 2 = 1–3 metastatic nodes, 3 = 4+ metastatic nodes) + histological grade (1 = good, 2 = moderate, 3 = poor).

A prognostic index < 3.4 = good prognosis, 3.4–5.4 = moderately good prognosis, >5.4 = poor prognosis.

Although many clinicians, particularly in the UK, rely on this method it still only produces a score for that patient's risk of relapse, and there is no universal agreement as to the cut-off level above which systemic therapy is indicated. So interpreting the answer from the formula, in terms of determining the treatment for a particular patient, is still a matter of personal judgement by the oncologists involved. 'Adjuvant on line' offers an alternative approach. Backed by a database from the National Cancer Institute in the USA this is an Internet service, which allows oncologists to enter the details of their patients and then to select a variety of adjuvant treatment options. The programme will then produce probable 5- and 10-year survival figures based on each treatment choice. This allows doctors to see which treatment is likely to be most effective and to get an estimate of the magnitude of the benefit. This system also provides data which are readily understood by patients, and so allows women to enter into a meaningful discussion with their oncologist in making treatment decisions.

When it comes to selecting which systemic therapy to use there have been a number of significant changes since the 1980s, including the following:

- The routine use of oestrogen receptor (ER) testing, and the realization that only those women with ER+ cancers will benefit from hormone therapy.
- The discovery of the aromatase inhibitors as an alternative to tamoxifen for post-menopausal women.
- The discovery of a number of new cytotoxic drugs which build on the benefits of the original CMF regime.
- The recognition that cytotoxic treatment is beneficial in post-menopausal women, and contributes to increased survival, although at a progressively diminishing level, up to the age of 70.
- The discovery of HER2 receptors and the recognition that women whose cancers are HER2+ may benefit from the addition of drugs like trastuzumab to their treatment regimen.

The discovery that only those women who had ER+ cancers would benefit from endocrine therapy initially simplified treatment decisions, but the advent of the aromatase inhibitors has complicated the picture. Clinical trial data suggest that these drugs are marginally more effective than tamoxifen in preventing relapse, perhaps reducing the risk of recurrence at 5 years by 3%–5%. Similar trials have also raised questions about the scheduling of hormonal therapy: traditionally tamoxifen has been given for 5 years but studies have shown that relapse rates can be reduced if either tamoxifen is given for 2–3 years followed by an aromatase inhibitor for 3 years or tamoxifen is given for 5 years followed by an aromatase inhibitor for a further 3 years. There are also issues around toxicity profile (a greater risk of menopausal symptoms, thromboembolic complications and endometrial hyperplasia and cancer, with tamoxifen, and osteoporosis, with aromatase inhibitors), and cost, with the aromatase inhibitors, being significantly more expensive than tamoxifen. At the present time there is no universal consensus on the optimum way to use endocrine therapy in early breast cancer and decisions will vary from oncologist to oncologist and patient to patient.

Other points to mention in relation to endocrine therapy relate to pre-menopausal women, and the sequencing of treatment. The aromatase inhibitors only work in post-menopausal women and, although tamoxifen may be used in younger women, its effect on ovarian function is variable and unpredictable. In the past when ovarian suppression was considered necessary the choice lay between surgical removal, oophorectomy, or radiotherapy, a radiation menopause. Nowadays, however, these have largely been supplanted by the use of injections of gonaderilin analogues, which offer long-term, but reversible prevention of oestrogen formation. The use of gonaderilin analogues in the adjuvant treatment of young women with breast cancer is variable. Some studies have suggested that they may be as effective as cytotoxic drugs, but they are seldom used as an alternative treatment. However, some oncologists will use them in addition to cytotoxics, particularly in women at high risk of relapse. In the past when an adjuvant treatment programme combined hormonal and cytotoxic therapy, the two modalities were usually given concurrently, but clinical trials have now shown that this reduces the effectiveness of cytotoxic treatment, and the pattern nowadays is to give cytotoxic therapy first, followed by hormonal manipulation. (The theoretical basis for the adverse interaction between endocrine and cytotoxic therapy is that the former reduces the level of cell division in the cancer, putting cells in the resting, G_o, phase of the cell cycle, where they are more resistant to cytotoxic treatment.) Incidentally, giving radiotherapy concurrently with cytotoxic treatment does not reduce its effectiveness, although side-effects, such as tiredness, may be increased.

When it comes to the choice of cytotoxic drug regimens for adjuvant therapy in early breast cancer there has been a similar evolutionary process. Clinical trials during the 1990s showed that the benefits of classical CMF chemotherapy could be increased by adding an anthracycline drug, usually epirubicin, to the combination. More recently trials have shown that combining epiribicin with the taxane, docetaxel, further increases the chance of cure. However, these additional benefits come at the cost of increased toxicity: for example, one major study with the epirubicin–docetaxel combination reported that 25% of women who had the drugs developed neutropenic sepsis. This means that in general oncologists will try and individualize the choice of treatment regimen for their patients, reserving the more aggressive drug combinations for women who are at high risk of relapse, and who are younger and fitter, whilst less intensive schedules are appropriate for older, frailer and lower risk women. Although studies have shown that cytotoxic treatment may have a positive impact on survival in women up to the age of 70, the benefit diminishes steadily over the age of 50 and so its use in women over 60 is, once again, a matter of weighing up the risks and benefits for individual patients. Over 70 the benefits are minimal, and the risk of significant toxicity increases dramatically, so cytotoxic treatment is seldom indicated.

For those women who have HER2+ cancers the addition of trastuzumab to their drug regimen has been shown to further reduce the risk of relapse. However, the extent of this benefit has been exaggerated by the media with an overall reduction of the relapse rate by only a matter of 2 or 3%. There is uncertainty of the duration of the necessary treatment, with initial studies suggesting giving the drug for 1–2 years, but later results have suggested that a treatment schedule as short as 4 months may be equally effective and carry a reduced risk of cardiotoxicity.

When it comes to the treatment of relapsed, metastatic, breast cancer the choice of systemic therapy depends on whether the tumour is ER+ or not, and whether there has been previous systemic adjuvant therapy. If the cancer is ER+ then hormonal therapy would usually be the first option, unless the disease appears particularly aggressive, when cytotoxics would be preferred. If an endocrine agent, such as tamoxifen or an aromatase inhibitor, has been given previously as adjuvant therapy, and if the disease-free interval to relapse has been more than a couple of years, then the same agent could be re-tested, for shorter intervals an alternative drug would usually be chosen. Once the cancer proves to no longer be responsive to hormonal manipulation, cytotoxics can be introduced, using similar drug regimens to those mentioned previously for adjuvant therapy.

Suggestions for further reading

Berry DA et al. Effect of screening and adjuvant therapy on mortality from breast cancer. New Engl J Med, 2005; 353: 1784–1792.

Early Breast Cancer Trialist's Collaborative Group (EBCTCG). Effects of chemotherapy and hormonal therapy for early breast cancer on recurrence and 15-year survival. Lancet, 2005; 365: 1687–1717.

Howell A. Adjuvant aromatase inhibitors for breast cancer. Lancet, 2005; 366: 431–433.

Smith IE, Chua S. Medical treatment of early breast cancer: 1. Adjuvant treatment. Br Med J, 2006; 332: 34–37.

Smith IE, Chua S. Medical treatment of early breast cancer: 2. Endocrine therapy. Br Med J, 2006; 332: 101–103.

NICE. TA112 Breast cancer (early) – hormonal treatment guidance., November 2006. www.nice.org.uk

Veronesi U, Boyle P, Goldhirsch A et al. Breast cancer. Lancet, 2005; 365: 1727–1741.

LUNG CANCER

Lung cancer is the second commonest cancer in UK. Each year there are more than 35,000 new cases, with some 32,000 people annually dying of the disease. More than 95% of lung cancers are smoking related. Although the incidence in men is decreasing that in women is still rising, giving a current male to female ratio of 3:2. The average age at the time of diagnosis is 65, with less than 2% of people being under the age of 50. Lung cancer can be divided into two main types: small cell lung cancer, which makes up about 20% of cases, and non-small cell lung cancer, which includes squamous carcinomas, adenocarcinomas and poorly differentiated carcinomas, and accounts for the remaining 80%. The management of these two forms of lung cancer is quite different.

Small Cell Lung Cancer
Small cell lung cancer can be classified as either limited, if the disease is confined to the hemithorax of origin and the mediastinum, or extensive, if there is spread elsewhere; 60–70% of people have extensive disease at the time of diagnosis. Until the 1970s both stages of the disease were uniformly rapidly fatal, with survival times being measured in a matter of weeks to a few months. The advent of intermittent combination cytotoxic chemotherapy dramatically transformed the outlook, as these tumours proved remarkably chemosensitive with about 80% of people going into remission, and about 20% experiencing complete remissions. Unfortunately this good news is offset by three negatives: firstly, most people will relapse; secondly, when relapse occurs second-line chemotherapy is rarely effective; and thirdly, despite numerous clinical trials with different drug regimens the results of treatment have hardly changed over the last 20 years.

A wide range of drug combinations have been found to be active in small cell lung cancer. These include etoposide and cisplatin (EC), and cyclophosphamide, doxorubicin and vincristine (CAV). No one regimen has been found to be significantly better than the rest. Overall use of one of these schedules will lead to average survival times of 18–24 months in people with limited-stage disease, and 7–12 months in those with extensive disease. Of those people with limited-stage disease about 15–20% will survive 5 years or more.

When good remissions were first seen following chemotherapy in small cell lung cancer one problem was that more than 50% of people relapsed with brain metastases. This was because the drugs used had little or no ability to penetrate the blood brain barrier, so seedlings of tumour that had lodged in the brain were able to continue growing. As a result 'prophylactic' radiotherapy to the brain was introduced for people who went into remission, and this is still widely used today as it reduces the CNS relapse rate by almost 50%. Radiotherapy to the primary site has also been advocated following chemotherapy for some patients with limited disease and may improve the chance of surviving 2 years or more by about 5%.

Non-small-Cell Lung Cancer

The cornerstone of treatment here for localized disease is surgery. Although this has the potential for cure, less than 10% of people are suitable for an operation, either because of the extent of their disease, their general fitness (many people will have severe respiratory or cardiac problems because of their chronic smoking) or their age. For some of these individuals, radical radiotherapy may be an alternative, but offers a lower chance of cure than surgery.

For many years there has been uncertainty as to whether giving adjuvant chemotherapy after apparently successful surgery would improve the outcome, but clinical trials reported in 2005 finally gave convincing evidence of a benefit. They showed that 5-year survival could be increased by about 15%, from around 50% to 58%. The treatment was based on either cisplatin and vinorelbine or taxotere and carboplatin, given for 4–6 courses over 4–6 months. There is still debate about the value of adjuvant chemotherapy in the earliest stages of the disease (stage 1A and B) but for people who have stage 2 or 3A tumours resected it is clearly indicated.

In people with advanced disease palliative, radiotherapy has been the mainstay of treatment for many years. Although this can offer effective symptom control, with cough, dyspnoea, chest pain and haemoptysis being relieved in more than 60% of cases, often by just one or two out-patient treatments, there is no effect on overall survival. In the late 1990s an overview of previous trials showed that platinum-based chemotherapy could increase life-expectancy, albeit only by a modest 6–8 weeks. Since that time, further trials have shown that a variety of regimens can extend survival by 4–5 months. But patient selection is an important issue. The chance of a benefit is strongly dependent on performance status, with fitter, younger people being the ones to benefit. As many patients are elderly or have very poor health due to smoking-related co-morbidities, this means that it is still probably a minority who are actually suitable for cytotoxic treatment.

First-line chemotherapy should usually be a combination of either cisplatin or carboplatin with either docetaxel, gemcitabine, paclitaxel or vinorelbine, taking account of the toxicities and convenience of the drugs in individual patients. Docetaxel as a monotherapy can be tried as second-line therapy on relapse.

The fact that 60% or more of non-small-cell lung cancers over express epidermal growth factor receptor (EGFR) means that in recent years there has been interest in the use of EGFR tyrosine kinase inhibitors in this disease. Two agents have been undergoing clinical trials: erlotinib and gefitinib. Looking at people who had relapsed after cytotoxic chemotherapy erlotinib extended survival by about 2 months, when compared to placebo, although the response rate was only about 10%. Once again, looking at relapse after cytotoxic treatment, initial trials with gefitinib were encouraging, but later results suggested that clear survival benefits were limited to non-smokers of Asian origin, but further studies may clarify these provisional findings.

Suggestions for further reading

Blackhall F, Thatcher N. Chemotherapy for advanced lung cancer. Eur J Oncol, 2004; 40: 2345–2348.

Doroshaw JH. Targeting EGFR in non-small cell lung cancer. New Engl J Med, 2005; 353: 200–202.

Jackman DM, Johnson BE. Small-cell lung cancer. Lancet 2005; 366: 1385–1397.

Silvestri GA, Spiro SG. Carcinoma of the bronchus 60 years later. Thorax 2006; 61: 1023–1028.

Pisters KMN. Adjuvant chemotherapy for non-small cell lung cancer – the smoke clears. N Engl J Med 2005; 352: 2640–2642.

NICE. Lung cancer: the diagnosis and treatment of lung cancer, quick reference guide. Clinical guideline 24. National Institute for Clinical Excellence, 2005.

MESOTHELIOMA

Mesothelioma is a primary cancer of the pleura (>90% of cases) or peritoneum. It is almost always related to previous asbestos exposure, often 30–40 years previously. There are some 2,000 new cases each year in UK, with a similar number of deaths. The incidence of mesothelioma is predicted to rise over the next few years to a peak, between 2010 and 2015. One estimate has suggested that during this period 1% of men born between 1940 and 1950 will die of the disease. Mesothelioma is much more common in men than women with a ratio of 6.5:1. The average age at diagnosis is 75. The overall 5-year survival is about 3%, with the median survival being about 9 months.

The very poor outcome for mesothelioma is in part due to the fact that it is usually only diagnosed at an advanced stage.

For those few patients where the disease is discovered sooner surgery, with an extrapleural pneumonectomy, may be an option. For most patients with more advanced disease, supportive care is often the only option but chemotherapy is occasionally given. In the past cisplatin and vinorelbine have been used as single agents, and mitomycin, vinblastine and cisplatin as a combination regimen. Although they produce occasional responses, none has been clearly shown to increase life-expectancy. Recently a trial combining pemetrexed and cisplatin with cisplatin alone showed that the two-drug schedule produced a higher response rate (41% versus 17%) and increased survival by about 3 months.

Suggestions for further reading
NICE. Mesothelioma – pemtrexed sodium: second appraisal consultation document. March 2007. www.nice.org.uk
Robinson BWS, Lake RA. Malignant mesothelioma. Lancet, 2005; 366: 397–408.
Tomek S, Emri S, Krejcy K, Manegold C. Chemotherapy for malignant pleural mesothelioma: past results and recent developments. Brit J Cancer, 2003; 88: 167–174.

UROLOGICAL CANCER

Kidney Cancer
There are 6,000 new cases of kidney cancer each year in UK, with just over 3,000 people annually dying of the disease. The average age at the time of diagnosis is 60. Renal cancer is twice as common in men than women. Smoking, obesity and hypertension all increase the risk of developing a renal cancer. Clear cell carcinomas account for more than 80% of renal cancers. Clear cell carcinoma of the kidney is a complication of the rare inherited syndrome von Hippel Lindau disease. The overall 5-year survival figure is 45%. This figure improving, partly because an increasing number of renal cancers, currently about 30%, are diagnosed as incidental findings in people having abdominal CT scans for some other reason, and hence are discovered at an early, pre-symptomatic, stage.

Surgery, with either a total or partial nephrectomy, is the definitive treatment for renal cancers. Adjuvant chemotherapy has nothing to offer. Historically chemotherapy has had a very limited role in advanced renal cancer. Cytotoxics have proved uniformly ineffective. The progestogen hormone Provera has been advocated but responses are rarely, if ever, seen. The cytokines interferon alpha and interleukin have been used but response rates are only of the order of 10%, with no good evidence of increased survival, and both drugs are associated with considerable toxicity (there is a geographical divide in the use of these two drugs, with interleukin being favoured in North America and interferon in Europe).

Recently attention has focused on angiogenesis inhibition. The background to this is that in von Hippel Lindau disease (VHL) the VHL tumour suppressor gene is inactivated. This same abnormality has now been identified in more than 60% of sporadic clear cell renal carcinomas. VHL inactivation leads to an increase in levels of vascular endothelial growth factor (VEGF), platelet derived growth factor α (PDGFα), and transforming growth factor a (TDGFα), all of which stimulate new blood vessel formation, and hence support tumour growth. Two drugs which appear to act primarily by inhibiting VEGF and PDGFα receptors have recently been approved for use in advanced renal cancer: sunitinib and sorafenib. Another drug temsirolimus acts at an earlier stage in the pathway by inhibiting production of VEGF and PDGF$^-\alpha$. All these agents are showing activity in patients with metastatic renal cancer but their impact on overall survival is still to be defined.

Suggestions for further reading
Brugarolas J. Renal-cell carcinoma – molecular pathways and therapies. New Engl J Med 2007; 356: 185–187.
Motzer RJ, Bukowski RM. Targeted therapies for metastatic renal cell carcinoma. J Clin Oncol 2006; 24: 5601–5608.

Bladder Cancer
Bladder cancer is the fifth commonest cancer in UK. There are about 14,000 new cases of bladder cancer each year, with 4,700 people dying annually of the disease. The average age at the time of diagnosis is 70. Bladder cancer is three times more common in men than women. Transitional cell carcinomas account for more than 90% of bladder cancers. The overall 5-year survival figure is 65%. This figure hides the fact that bladder cancer is made up of two different types of disease: superficial and invasive cancers.

Superficial bladder cancers are tumours confined to the mucosal lining of the bladder. They make up 70% of bladder cancers. Based on the microscopic appearance of the tumour cells they can be classified as low-risk or high-risk cancers. Low-risk cancers, which account for 60% of superficial tumours, behave in a relatively benign way. High-risk cancers carry the risk of transformation to invasive disease. Management of these growths is by an initial cystoscopic resection, or diathermy of the cancer, followed immediately by instillation of a chemical into the bladder. The drug is introduced through a catheter at the time of operation, the catheter is then clamped for the next few hours allowing the drug to be partly absorbed by the bladder wall. For low-risk tumours all that is then required is a regular follow up cystoscopy to check that there is no evidence of recurrence. For high-risk tumours similar regular cystoscopies are offered but are usually followed by further drug instillations. For some patients with extensive high-risk disease, where there is considered to be a very strong chance of invasive cancer developing, a radical cystectomy may be offered as an alternative.

The most widely used, and most effective, chemical for bladder instillations is Bacille Calmette-Guerin (BCG), which was for many years used as a vaccine against tuberculosis. Quite why it is so effective in treating superficial bladder cancer remains uncertain. Solutions of a number of cytotoxic drugs may be used as an alternative to BCG; among the drugs used are mitomycin, epirubicin and doxorubicin.

For invasive cancers surgery is the cornerstone of treatment, with a radical cystectomy being offered. As bladder cancer is mainly a disease of older people, many patients will not be fit enough for major surgery and radiotherapy is the treatment of choice for them. Unfortunately 5-year survival rates are poor: about 35% after surgery, and 25% after radiotherapy. Giving adjuvant chemotherapy after surgery does not significantly improve these figures. However, a number of trials have used a variety of cisplatin-based regimens given pre-operatively (neo-adjuvant therapy) and have shown an overall increase in survival of about 5% and this may be offered as a treatment option for fitter patients.

For people with advanced or metastatic bladder cancer, chemotherapy has a limited role. The most widely used cytotoxic regimen is M-VAC (methotrexate, vinblastine, doxorubicin and cisplatin). More recently the combination of gemcitabine and cisplatin has been advocated as a less toxic alternative. These combinations give response rates of about 40% and may increase survival by 4–6 months. It has recently been recognized that up to 50% of bladder cancers over-express HER2, and so might be susceptible to agents like trastuzumab. There is also interest in evaluating drugs reducing VEGF or inhibiting VEGF receptors. These prospects remains to be explored.

Suggestions for further reading
Bellmont J, Albiol S. Chemotherapy for metastatic bladder cancer. Semin Oncol, 2007; 34: 135–144.

Garcia JA, Dreicer R. Systemic chemotherapy for advanced bladder cancer: update and controversies. J Clin Oncol 2006; 24: 5545–5551.

Parekh DJ, Bochner BH, Dalbagni G. Superficial and muscle-invasive bladder cancer: principles of management for outcome assessments. J Clin Oncol 2006; 24: 5519–5527.

Sternberg CN. Perioperative chemotherapy in muscle invasive bladder cancer to enhance survival or as a strategy for bladder preservation. Semin Oncol, 2007; 34: 122–128.

Prostate Cancer

Prostate cancer is the fourth commonest cancer in UK and has recently overtaken lung cancer as the commonest cancer in men. There are more than 32,000 new cases of prostate cancer each year, with some 8,500 men dying annually of the disease. Between 1990 and 2002 the annual age-adjusted incidence of prostate cancer nearly doubled in the UK. This was probably largely due to the availability of the prostate specific antigen (PSA) blood test, which allows the condition to be diagnosed at an early, asymptomatic stage, rather than a true increase in the frequency of prostate cancer. The average age at the time of diagnosis is 70–75. Increasing age is the greatest risk factor for developing prostate cancer, and it has been estimated that almost 100% of men in their 90s will have the disease. In younger men, in their 50s and 60s the disease tends to behave aggressively whereas in older men, in their 70s and 80s, it is often indolent, progressing very slowly, causing few problems and needing little or no treatment. Prostate cancers are adenocarcinomas and are graded according to their Gleason score, which ranges from 6 to 10, higher scores indicating more aggressive disease and a poorer prognosis. When prostate cancer spreads to other parts of the body it almost invariably goes to the bones. The overall 5-year survival rate is 71%.

When considering its management prostate cancer can be divided into three stages:

1. Early disease: when the cancer is confined within the capsule of the prostate gland.
2. Locally advanced disease: when the tumour has breached the capsule and spread into the surrounding tissues or pelvic lymph nodes.
3. Advanced disease: when blood-borne spread to the bones has occurred.

About 50% of men will present with early disease, 25% with locally advanced disease, and 25% with metastatic disease.

Options for the management of early prostate cancer include radical prostatectomy, radiotherapy (which may be either external beam – conformal or intensity modulated, IMRT, irradiation – or brachytherapy, with the insertion of radioactive seeds into the prostate gland), or a policy of watchful waiting. The latter is most appropriate for older mean (with a life-expectancy of 10 years or less) who have few symptoms, for whom treatment can be reserved until there is clear evidence of disease progression with either a rapidly rising PSA or symptoms developing. For younger men the results of either surgery or irradiation are similar.

A key question is whether giving hormonal therapy in addition to these other treatment modalities can improve the outcome. Studies are still ongoing, but the early evidence is that there may be a benefit, particularly in combination with radiotherapy. Practice is evolving in this area, but in the UK adjuvant endocrine therapy is being used increasingly, especially for those men deemed likely to have more aggressive tumours (those of younger age, or who have cancers with higher Gleason scores, or a higher PSA level). The optimum timing of treatment (whether started before or after surgery or radiotherapy) and its duration (anywhere from 2 months to 2 years) remain to be confirmed. Therapy usually involves either a gonadorelin analogue (such as goserelin, or leuprorelin), or an anti-androgen (such as bicalutamide, or flutamide).

For locally advanced prostate cancer the options are either external beam radiotherapy (the extent of disease means brachytherapy is not appropriate), or endocrine therapy, or, more usually nowadays, a combination of the two.

Since the mid-1940s endocrine therapy has been the cornerstone of management of advanced prostate cancer. Initially the options were a bilateral subcapsular orchidectomy, or the use of oral stilboestrol. Later it was discovered that stilboestrol carried a significantly increased risk of thromboembolic complications and was displaced by the newer anti-androgens and gonadorelin analogues (although it is still sometimes used as a third- or fourth-line therapy). Although it may seem somewhat barbaric, castration, with an orchidectomy, is still the treatment which some older men prefer, feeling that it spares them anxiety of having to remember to take medication, and may carry fewer side-effects. Otherwise the choice is between either a gonadorelin analogue or an anti-androgen. Once the first-line therapy is no longer controlling the disease then whichever type of drug was not used initially can be substituted.

Traditionally hormone therapy has been given continuously for men with metastatic prostate cancer but recently it has been suggested that treatment might be equally, or even more, effective, if given on an intermittent basis. Clinical trials using various schedules have indicated that this might be the case, and even if there is no actual survival advantage then the time off-treatment has benefits in terms of quality of life of patients and the overall cost of treatment, so this approach is increasingly entering into routine practice.

Combining a gonadorelin analogue and an anti-androgen has been evaluated, the approach being known as total androgen blockade. Overall trials suggest that there is no advantage to giving the drugs together rather than sequencing the therapies. If, however, a man who has never had endocrine therapy is to be given a gonadorelin analogue then he should also have an anti-androgen for the first 2–3 weeks of treatment since sometimes the gonadorelin analogues can cause a surge of androgen release, before inhibition, which can lead to a sudden increase in symptoms known as a tumour flare.

Apart from stilboestrol another option for third- or fourth-line treatment is the use of corticosteroids. Both prednisolone and dexamethesone may bring about further worthwhile responses.

Until a few years ago it was widely agreed that cytotoxic therapy played little or no part in the treatment of advanced prostate cancer. But in 2005 studies were published showing that regimens based around docetaxel could actually lead to an increase in survival, even though the median figure was less than 2 months. Although this is a modest benefit, there is also evidence that giving cytotoxic therapy with docetaxel may also help with symptom control and improve quality of life of many men.

Suggestions for further reading

Collins R, Trowman R, Norman G et al. A systematic review of the effectiveness of docetaxel and mitoxantrone for the treatment of metastatic hormone-refractory prostate cancer. Br J Cancer, 2006; 95: 457–462.

Heidenreich A, Aus G, Abbou CC et al. European Association of Urology: guidelines on prostate cancer, 2007. www.uroweb.org

Loblaw DA, Virgo KS, Nam R et al. Initial hormonal management of androgen-sensitive metastatic, recurrent, or progressive prostate cancer: 2006 update of an American Society of Clinical Oncology Practice Guideline. J Clin Oncol, 2007; 25: 1596–1605.

Testicular Cancer

There are more than 1,800 new cases of testicular cancer each year in UK. Although this is a relatively small number, it is the commonest form of cancer in men under 45, with an average age of onset of 30. The incidence of testicular cancer has doubled in the last 40 years and is still rising at 3%–6% per annum. The reason for this increase is unknown. Testicular cancers are classified as either seminomas (which make up 55% of all cases) or non-seminomatous cancers, a group made up of various forms of teratoma (30% of all cases) or mixed teratomas and seminomas (15%). Seminomas and teratomas are collectively known as germ-cell cancers of the testis. Surgery, with removal of the affected testis is the first line of treatment. Testicular cancer has been a major success story for cytotoxic chemotherapy; 50 years ago metastatic disease was universally fatal but today, even for men with poor prognosis secondary disease, two out of three can expect to be cured, and the overall cure rate for testicular cancer is in excess of 95%.

In the past radiotherapy to the para-aortic and ipsilateral iliac lymph nodes was offered as standard adjuvant therapy for men with early stage seminomas. Later trials have shown that low-dose radiotherapy confined to the para-artic nodes is adequate and causes less long-term morbidity. Recently trials have also shown that a single course of the cytotoxic carboplatin is equivalent to irradiation. So currently the options for management are surveillance only, para-aortic radiotherapy or carboplatin. If the disease has spread to the iliac or para-aortic nodes, then irradiation plus carboplatin is recommended. Treatment with three courses of BEP cytotoxic chemotherapy (see below) is the standard of care for metastatic disease.

The management of non-seminomatous cancers was transformed by the introduction of the BEP regimen in the 1970s. This comprises the three drugs, bleomycin, etoposide and cisplatin. After an orchidectomy to remove the primary cancer 25–30% of men with early stage disease will relapse. Options for their management are close surveillance, with regular scans and measurements of tumour markers, offering treatment only when relapse is apparent, or a para-aortic lymph node dissection plus chemotherapy, or two courses of BEP chemotherapy. For men who have metastatic disease the definitive treatment is four courses of BEP.

As present outcomes are so good the main focus for future development is the search for less toxic treatment regimens which will minimize the risk of long-term side effects.

Suggestions for further reading
de Wit R, Fizazi K. Controversies in the management of clinical stage I testis cancer. J Clin Oncol, 2006; 24: 5482–5492.

Horwich A, Shipley J, Huddart R. Testicular germ-cell cancer. Lancet, 2005; 367: 754–765.

Kondagunta GV, Motzer RJ. Chemotherapy for advanced germ cell tumors. J Clin Oncol, 2006; 24: 5493–5502.

GASTROINTESTINAL CANCER

Oesophageal Cancer

Oesophageal cancer is the ninth commonest cancer in UK. There are about 7,500 new cases of oesophageal cancer each year, with some 6,500 people dying annually of the disease. The average age at the time of diagnosis is 72. Cancers of the upper and middle third of the oesophagus are usually squamous carcinomas whereas those of the lower third are adenocarcinomas. Squamous cancers used to be the more common of the two, but in recent years the incidence of adenocarcinomas has been increasing and these now account for half of all oesophageal cancers. Overall cancer of the oesophagus is about twice as common in men than women, but adenocarcinomas are five times more common in men. The overall 5-year survival figure in the UK is 8%.

For people with localized squamous carcinomas of the upper third of the oesophagus, chemoradiotherapy has increasingly taken over from surgery as the treatment of choice in recent years. The most widely used drug regimen in this situation is a combination of cisplatin and fluorouracil. For early carcinomas of the middle and lower third, surgery is usually recommended but in recent years it has been shown that giving pre-operative (neoadjuvant) chemotherapy can improve the outcome, the chemotherapy regimens used usually being based on either cisplatin and fluorouracil or cisplatin and bleomycin for squamous carcinomas, and epirubicin and cisplatin with continuous infusion of fluorouracil for adencoarcinomas. In the latter instance the drugs are continued for some weeks after surgery.

For some frailer patients with early disease of the middle or lower oesophagus chemoradiation appears to be an effective alternative to surgery. For more locally advanced cancers chemoradiation has been shown to produce transient complete responses in about two-thirds of patients with an overall increase in survival of about 6 months. For patients with advanced disease chemotherapy has been shown to increase survival by 4–6 months, with similar regimens to those used for neoadjuvant therapy. More recently other drugs are being evaluated, with capecitabine as a possible alternative to fluorouracil and oxali-platin instead of cisplatin. Paclitaxel has also shown some promise in these tumours, as has the monoclonal antibody bevacizumab.

Despite the encouraging improvements in outcome with the greater use of chemotherapy in recent years, it must be remembered that many of these figures come from clinical trials, which have included younger fitter patients. Unfortunately many people with oesophageal cancer are still too old and frail when their diagnosis is made to allow anything more than good supportive care, to maximize their quality of life in their terminal illness.

Suggestions for further reading

Allum WH, Griffin SM, Watson A et al. Guidelines on the management of oesophageal and gastric cancer. Gut 2002, 50 Supplement V: 1–21.

ESMO. Minimum clinical recommendations for diagnosis, treatment and follow-up of oesophageal cancer. Annals Oncol, 2005; 16 (supplement 1): i26–i27.

Munro AJ. Oesophageal cancer: an overview of overviews. Lancet, 2004; 364: 566–568.

Stomach Cancer

There are about 8,500 new cases of stomach cancer each year in UK, making it the seventh commonest cancer. Unlike many other cancers, the incidence of gastric cancer is decreasing, the numbers in the UK having halved over the last 30 years. Some 5,500 people die annually of the disease. The average age at the time of diagnosis is in the early 70s. Cancer of the stomach is more common in men than women with a ratio of 5:3. The overall 5-year survival figure in the UK is 15%.

Surgery is the cornerstone of treatment for gastric cancer but unfortunately only a minority of patients have operable disease at the time of their presentation. Studies of post-operative adjuvant chemotherapy have been done over the last 25 years but there is no convincing evidence of a benefit. However, two recent trials using different approaches have shown some promise, with a modest improvement in overall survival. In the one pre-operative treatment, with cisplatin, epirubicin and fluorouracil was followed by the same three drugs being given post-operatively, in the other chemoradiation, using fluorouracil and leucovorin as the cytotoxic treatment, was given post-operatively. In advanced disease the cisplatin, epirubicin and fluorouracil regimen has been the most widely used and does produce responses in up to 60% of patients with an increase in survival of 4–6 months. As with oesophageal adenocarcinomas other drugs are being evaluated, with capecitabine as a possible alternative to fluorouracil and oxaliplatin instead of cisplatin. In addition irinotecan, paclitaxel and docetaxel have all shown good response rates and are being assessed in a number of different treatment schedules.

Suggestions for further reading
Allum WH, Griffin SM, Watson A et al. Guidelines on the management of oesophageal and gastric cancer. Gut 2002; 50 Supplement V: 1–21.

Wagner AD, Grothe W, Haerting J et al. Chemotherapy in advanced gastric cancer: a systematic review and meta-analysis. J Clin Oncol, 2006; 24: 2903–2909.

Lim L, Michael M, Mann GB et al. Review article: adjuvant therapy in gastric cancer. J Clin Oncol, 2005; 23: 6220–6232.

Carcinoma of the Pancreas
There are about 7,000 new cases of pancreatic cancer each year in UK, making it the tenth commonest cancer. About 6,400 people die annually from the disease. The average age at the time of diagnosis is in the early 70s. Cancer of the pancreas is equally common in both sexes. The overall 5-year survival figure in the UK is 2% and most people survive less than 6 months.

Surgical resection offers the only hope of cure but less than 1 in 10 patients will have operable disease and even then the 5-year survival rate is only of the order of 10%. Clinical trials have looked at both adjuvant chemotherapy and adjuvant chemoradiation to try and improve these figures. The chemotherapy regimens have been based on fluorouracil, most often combined with either mitomycin or doxorubicin. Adjuvant chemotherapy seems to be of some value, possibly increasing 5-year survival from about 10% to about 20%, but overall chemoradiation does not seem to be beneficial.

Many people with advanced pancreatic cancer will be too ill, and will deteriorate too rapidly, for chemotherapy to be considered. For those patients who are considered for treatment, fluorouracil was the drug of choice for many years, but the results were disappointing. More recently gemcitabine has been shown to be superior to fluorouracil, with some studies showing 1-year survival increased to 20% compared to less than 5% with fluorouracil, together with a measurable improvement in quality of life. As a result of these modestly encouraging findings the drug is now being assessed in the adjuvant setting. Combining gemcitabine with a number of other cytotoxics in advanced disease is also being explored, with fluorouracil, docetaxel, cisplatin, oxaliplatin and irinotecan all being evaluated. There is also some evidence that the monoclonal antibodies cetuximab and trastuzumab may have a role to play.

Suggestions for further reading

Li D, Keping X, Wolff R, Abbruzzese JL. Pancreatic cancer. Lancet, 2004; 363: 1049–1057.

Stocken DD, Buchler MW, Dervenis C et al . Meta-analysis of randomised adjuvant trials for pancreatic cancer. Br J Cancer 2005, 92: 1372–1381.

Colorectal Cancer

Colorectal cancer is the third commonest cancer in UK. There are more than 34,000 new cases of colorectal cancer each year, with 17,000 people dying annually of the disease. There are about 22,000 new case of colon cancer and about 12,000 of rectal cancer each year. The average age at the time of diagnosis is 70. Colon cancer is equally common in men and women but rectal cancer occurs more often in men with a male to female ratio of 3:2. Most colorectal cancers are thought to arise from pre-existing polyps in the wall of the bowel and about 4% are due to the inherited conditions familial polyposis coli or hereditary non-polyposis coli (these account for most of the cases in younger age groups). Wherever possible, surgery is the cornerstone of treatment. The overall 5-year survival figure in the UK for both colonic and rectal cancer is 50%.

In the 1950s fluorouracil was identified as the only cytotoxic drug to have any significant activity in colorectal cancer, but even so response rates were disappointing with only about 1 in 10 people with advanced disease seeing a benefit. In the 1970s the addition of folinic acid (leucovorin), which prolongs the inhibition of fluorouracil's target enzyme, thymidylate synthase, brought about an improvement with response rates in metastatic disease rising to about 30%. Over the next decade a lot of work went into exploring different schedules of administration of the two drugs to maximize their efficacy. Regimens which evolved included low-dose folinic acid and bolus injections of fluorouracil (Mayo), high-dose folinic acid, bolus and infusion of fluorouracil (de Gramont) and prolonged intravenous infusion of fluorouracil (Lokich). During this time clinical trials also showed that the drugs had some activity as adjuvant therapy in earlier stages of the disease. In the mid-1990s three further active cytotoxics were introduced, irinotecan, oxaliplatin and the oral drug capecitabine, which is similar to fluorouracil in its mode of action. More recently two monoclonal antibodies have also shown some promise in the treatment of bowel cancer, these are bevacizumab and cetuximab. With so many recent developments the role of chemotherapy in colorectal cancer is still evolving, and the optimum management is for patients to go into clinical trials whenever possible.

In stage III colon cancer, when the disease has reached local lymph nodes but there is no obvious distant spread, adjuvant chemotherapy is generally recommended for patients under the age of 70 (although often given, the value of adjuvant chemotherapy in people over 70 is uncertain and controversial). By using fluorouracil- and leucovorin-based regimens, an increase in 5-year survival of about 10% can be expected. Newer regimens adding oxaliplatin to these drugs, or giving oral capecitabine, suggest a modest improvement on this figure may be possible, but long-term trial results are still awaited. For people with stage II colon cancer the benefit of adjuvant chemotherapy is less certain, with perhaps a 5% improvement in 5-year survival, and guidelines suggest it should be reserved for those patients who are considered to be at high risk of recurrence. Incidentally, the 'Adjuvant on line' service (mentioned in the section on Breast Cancer, p. 79) is also programmed for colorectal cancer, to help clinicians, and patients decide on the whether treatment is appropriate, and which agents should be given.

In stage II and III rectal cancer the focus has been on combining chemotherapy and radiation. Post-operative chemoradiation, using fluorouracil and leucovorin, has been shown to reduce local recurrence rates and improve long-term survival. With the introduction of routine MRI scanning to accurately stage tumours pre-operatively it has been possible to clearly identify those cancers which are locally advanced and for these pre-operative chemoradiation is increasingly being offered. This neo-adjuvant therapy can lead to a complete response rate of about 20%, with no trace of the tumour being detectable at surgery. Trials are beginning to explore the incorporation of the newer drugs into these treatment schedules, but as yet no results are available.

In metastatic colorectal cancer the optimum management has still to be defined. Most bowel cancers spread to the liver, and when the disease is localized within the liver surgical resection of metastases may result in a cure. The criteria for considering surgery are widening all the time but at present about 15% of people with liver secondaries are elligible for surgery and of these about 30–35% will survive 5 years or more. Increasingly chemotherapy is being used pre-operatively to shrink the size and number of liver secondaries which further increases the number of patients for whom resection is possible and improves the outcome.

For people with metastatic disease for whom there is no possibility of hepatic resection survival averages 9–10 months. Giving fluorouracil–leucovorin chemotherapy increases this to an average of 12 months. Early studies adding oxaliplatin (the FOLFOX regimen) showed life expectancy extended to a median of about 15 months but later studies, using modified drug doses and scheduling, are reporting average survivals of 20 months or more. The incorporation of irinotecan or capecitabine into these regimens is also being explored. Recently, however, there has been great interest in the use of the monoclonal antibodies, bevacizumab or cetuximab. The data on these agents is limited but early results have suggested they may result in a further increase in survival when added to conventional cytotoxic regimens. The expense of such regimens is, however, very considerable, and for the moment they are considered non-cost effective until stronger evidence of a benefit emerges from ongoing trials.

Suggestions for further reading

Bendell J. Optimum chemotherapy for metastatic colorectal cancer. Lancet, 2006; 368: 2039–2040.

Benson AH, Schrag D, Somerfield MR et al. American Society of Clinical Oncology recommendations on adjuvant chemotherapy for stage II colon cancer. J Clin Oncol, 2004; 22: 3408–3419.

NICE. Final appraisal determination: bevacizumab and cetuximab for metastatic colorectal cancer. August 2006. www.nice.org.uk.

Saletti P, Cavalli F. Metastatic colorectal cancer. Cancer Treat Rev, 2006; 32: 557–571.

Wertz J, Koch M, Debus J et al. Colorectal cancer. Lancet, 2005; 365: 153–165.

GYNAECOLOGICAL CANCER

Cancer of the Ovary

There are about 7,000 new cases of ovarian cancer each year in UK, with nearly 4,500 women dying annually of the disease. It is the fourth commonest cancer in women. The average age at the time of diagnosis is 70. There are many different histological types of cancer of the ovary but the great majority are adenocarcinomas, arising from the serosal surface of the organ; this summary focuses on these tumours. The overall 5-year survival figure in the UK is about 35%.

The first line of treatment for ovarian cancer is surgery, with removal of both ovaries, the fallopian tubes and uterus. Even when the growth has spread into the peritoneal cavity surgery is still recommended, with as much of the metastatic disease as possible being removed (debulking surgery). For those women with very early disease, where the tumour is well differentiated and confined to one ovary, no further treatment is indicated but for all others the standard of care is adjuvant cytotoxic chemotherapy. For women with poorly differentiated cancer confined to one ovary this may be carboplatin as a single agent but for all others it should be six courses of a platinum and taxane based combination.

Another approach to post-surgical chemotherapy is the addition of intraperitoneal drug administration, via a catheter through the abdominal wall, into the peritoneal cavity. A number of regimens have been used. One of the most recent, and most successful, involved giving conventional courses of intravenous cisplatin and paclitaxel, followed by intraperitoneal cisplatin 2 and 8 days later. Whilst this did lead to a prolongation of overall survival, compared to intravenous chemotherapy alone, it did cause a considerable increase in toxicity. At present intraperitoneal chemotherapy remains an essentially experimental treatment for ovarian cancer.

Ovarian cancer is chemosensitive and even with advanced disease about 75% of women will gain a remission. However, after about 18–24 months most will relapse with recurrent disease. At this stage treatment depends on their response to first-line chemotherapy, which falls into four categories:

1. Platinum-sensitive disease: This is a cancer that responds to first-line platinum-based chemotherapy and relapses more than 12 months after completion of that therapy.
2. Partially platinum-sensitive disease: This is a cancer that initially responds to platinum-based chemotherapy but relapses between 6 and 12 months after treatment has been completed.
3. Platinum-resistant disease: This is where the cancer responds initially but relapses within 6 months of completing platinum-based chemotherapy.
4. Platinum-refractory disease: This is where the cancer does not respond at all to platinum-based chemotherapy.

For women with platinum-sensitive, or partially platinum-sensitive, disease then a further trial of either cisplatin or carboplatin, combined with paclitaxel, is recommended. For women with platinum-resistant, or platinum-refractory, disease single-agent paclitaxel can be tried. An alternative second-line (or subsequent) treatment for partially platinum-sensitive, platinum-resistant or platinum-refractory disease is the liposomal form of doxorubicin: pegylated liposomal doxorubicin. Another option for the latter two groups is single-agent topotecan therapy.

About 50% of ovarian cancers over express EGFR and early studies suggest that EGFR tyrosine kinase inhibitors, such as erlotinib, may be of value for some women. Similarly studies are underway looking at anti-angiogenesis agents, such as bevac-uzimab, and these are also showing some promise. It is too early to say whether the use of these targeted-therapies will have a significant impact on the management of women with ovarian cancer.

Suggestions for further reading
Cannistra SA. Cancer of the ovary. N Engl J med, 2004; 351: 2519–2529.
ESMO. Minimum clinical recommendations for diagnosis, treatment and follow-up of epithelial ovarian cancer. Annals Oncol, 2005; 16 (supplement 1): i13–i15.
Markman M, Walker JL. Intraperitoneal chemotherapy of ovarian cancer: a review, with a focus on practical aspects of treatment. J Clin Oncol, 2006; 24: 988–994.

Cervical Cancer
There are about 3,100 new cases of invasive cervical cancer each year in UK, with 1,200 women dying annually of the disease. It is the seventh commonest cancer in women. The disease can appear any time after the age of 20 and there are two peaks of incidence at about 40 and in the early 70s. Of cervical cancers, 70% are squamous carcinomas, 15% are adenocarcinomas and the remainder are mixed tumours. The overall 5-year survival figure in the UK is about 65%.

The treatment of invasive cervical cancer is stage dependent. For early disease (stages Ib to IIa) radical surgery and radical radiotherapy are equally effective, leading to a cure for about 90% of women. For locally advanced disease (stages IIb to IVa) chemoradiation is generally the preferred treatment. The most successful drug in this context has been cisplatin, and a number of clinical trials have shown that combining it with radiation increases survival from about 60% to 80%, when compared with radiotherapy alone. To try and improve on these figures newer trials are looking at combining other cytotoxics with cisplatin, candidate drugs include paclitaxel and gemcitabine. The success of chemoradiation in bulky cervical cancer has led some clinicians to use it in earlier stage disease, either as an alternative or as an adjunct to surgery.

For recurrent or advanced cervical cancer cisplatin has shown activity when used as a single agent, giving response rates of about 20%. To try and improve on this studies have been done combining cisplatin with either paclitaxel or topotecan. Both combinations increased the response rate to about 35%. However, there is little evidence that chemotherapy increases overall survival, which averages about 10 months. Other drugs that have recently shown activity in cervical cancer are gemcitabine and vinorelbine and clinical trials are underway looking at these agents in combination with cisplatin.

Although they do not fall strictly under the heading of chemotherapy, it is important to mention that two vaccines are now available to protect against cervical cancer. More than 95% of cervical cancers are linked to human papilloma virus (HPV) infection, and about 70% are specifically linked to the type 16 and 18 HPV virus. Two vaccines, Gardasil and Cervarix, have been developed against HPV 16 and 18 and their recent availability offers the possibility of a dramatic reduction in cervical cancer incidence over the coming decades.

Suggestions for further reading

Kesic V. Management of cervical cancer. Eur J Surg Oncol, 2006; 32: 832–837.

Lowndes CM, Gill ON. Cervical cancer, human papilloma virus and vaccination. Br Med J, 2005; 331: 915–916.

Moore D. Chemotherapy for recurrent cervical cancer. Curr Opinion Oncol, 2006; 18: 516-9

Rojas-Espaillat LA, Rose PG. Management of locally advanced cervical cancer. Curr Opin Oncol, 2005; 17: 485–492.

Tzioras S, Paulidis N, Paraskevaidis E, Ioannidis JPA. Effects of different chemotherapy regimens on survival for advanced cervical cancer: systematic review and meta analysis. Cancer Treat Rev, 2007; 33: 24–38.

Uterine Cancer

There are about 4,500 new cases of cancer of the womb each year in UK, with 900 women dying annually of the disease. It is the fifth commonest cancer in women. The disease is rare before the age of 40 but rises rapidly in incidence between 40 and 50 remaining relatively constant thereafter until the age of 80, when its frequency declines. More than 85% of uterine cancers are adenocarcinomas arising from the endometrial lining of the organ. The remainder are either squamous cell carcinomas or uterine sarcomas. Between 70% and 80% of endometrial adeno-carcinomas will be positive for progesterone receptors (PgR+), these are more likely to be present in well-differentiated tumours. The overall 5-year survival figure in the UK is about 76%.

The first-line treatment for endometrial adenocarcinomas is surgery, which will usually involve a hysterectomy and bilateral salpingo-oophorectomy. Practice varies, but this is commonly followed by adjuvant radiotherapy to the pelvis. A number of clinical trials have failed to show any clear benefit for adjuvant hormonal or cytotoxic therapy.

For women with advanced or relapsed disease, hormonal treatment with progestogens, such as medroxyprogesterone acetate or megestrol acetate, is often worthwhile and can lead to quite long-lasting remissions. For hormone-resistant cancers cytotoxic therapy is an option. Studies have shown that the combination of cisplatin and doxorubicin produces responses in about one-third of women, and the addition of paclitaxel may raise this figure to over 50%. However, there is no clear evidence that cytotoxic therapy actually increases survival, and so using a less-toxic regimen may be preferable, especially as one is often dealing with an older population.

Suggestion for further reading
Carey MS, Gawlik, C, Fung-Kee M et al. Systematic overview of systemic therapy for advanced or recurrent endometrial cancer. Gynecol Oncol, 2006; 101: 158–167.

BRAIN TUMOURS
Primary brain tumours make up about 1% of all cancers. They are a very diverse group of malignancies. Numerically the gliomas dominate (these are tumours arising from the supportive tissues within the brain, rather than neural tissue). Of the gliomas by far the most common are the astrocytomas, with nearly 4,000 new cases in adults each year in UK, and about 3,000 deaths each year. Astrocytomas are also the commonest of all solid tumours in children. In adults the incidence of astrocytomas increases progressively with age, the average age at diagnosis being about 57. Astrocytomas are classified according to their histological appearance into either low-grade (Grades I and II) or high-grade (Grades III and IV) lesions. Grade III lesions are also known as anaplastic astrocytomas and grade IV astrocytomas are also known as glioblastoma multiforme. Low-grade astrocytomas behave in a relatively benign fashion, and chemotherapy plays little or no part in their management. High-grade astrocytomas,

which account for more than 60% of these tumours, behave much more aggressively and carry a poor prognosis. Age is a strong predictor of outcome for high-grade tumours, with about 50% of those under 40 surviving 18 months or more, whereas for people over 60 the figure less than 10%. The overall 5-year survival is less than 5%.

With their aggressive behaviour and frequent rapid deterioration, many people with high-grade astrocytomas, especially the elderly and those with a poor performance status, are not candidates for active treatment.

Many patients get dramatic short-term symptomatic relief from high-dose steroid therapy (dexamethasone, up to 16mg daily) and for many people this, combined with general supportive care, is the most appropriate treatment. For younger fitter patients surgery is often considered, but even when performed it is usually only possible to debulk the tumour rather than remove it completely. In this situation implantation of Gliadel wafers at the time of operation may improve the outcome. These Gliadel implants are disc-shaped gel wafers, about 1cm in diameter. They contain the cytotoxic carmustine, and slowly dissolve in the brain, releasing the drug into the surrounding tissues over a period of 2–3 weeks.

For most patients who have surgery this will be followed by radiotherapy to the brain, and radiotherapy is also the treatment option for those patients who were not suitable for surgery but are still fit enough for active treatment to be considered. Studies have suggested that adjuvant chemotherapy may be of value in selected patients, increasing survival by 2–3 months, and the two regimes that have been most widely used in the past are lomustine (CCNU), as a single agent, and PCV (procarbazine, lomustine and vincrtistine), more recently temozolamide is being increasingly used. There is also evidence that giving temozolamide in combination with radiotherapy, and continuing the drug thereafter, improves the survival by about 6 months, when compared to radiation alone. For patients who relapse, or have progressive disease, after radiotherapy, and have not previously had temozolamide this is now supplanting lomustine as the first-line treatment. Temozolamide is also being increasingly used as the first-line chemotherapy for fitter patients, with a good performance status.

Suggestions for further reading
NICE. Glioma (newly diagnosed high-grade) – carmustine implants and temozolamide: consultation appraisal document. December 2006. www.nice.org.uk

Stupp R, Mason WP, van den Baent MJ et al. Radiotherapy plus concomitant and adjuvant temozolamide for glioblastoma. New Engl J Med, 2005; 352: 986–996.

HEAD AND NECK CANCER

In UK there are nearly 9,000 new cases of head and neck cancer each year, with some 2,700 deaths. Head and neck cancers comprise a very diverse group of tumours, but more than 80% are squamous cell carcinomas of the oral cavity, oropharynx or larynx. This discussion will be restricted to these lesions. They occur more often in men than women, at a ratio of 2.5:1. The average age at diagnosis is around 65. The overall 5-year survival rate for squamous cell cancers of the oral cavity and oropharynx is about 47%, whilst that for laryngeal cancers is about 65%.

Head and neck cancer is one area in oncology where the role of chemotherapy is developing particularly rapidly. This constantly evolving situation means that there are no universally agreed guidelines and practice is likely to vary quite significantly from centre to centre. As far as first-line treatment is concerned either surgery or radiotherapy maybe appropriate depending on factors such as the site and size of the tumour and the general fitness of the patient.

In recent years clear evidence has emerged that the results of radiotherapy can be improved by giving concurrent chemotherapy (chemoradiation), particularly in people with locally advanced disease. This does, however, increase the risk of severe side effects and so is generally avoided for those with very early stage disease (where less intensive treatment is still effective), or those who are less fit or who have metastatic disease. Cisplatin is the most widely used cytotoxic in combination with radiation. But a recent development is the discovery that combining the EGFR antagonist, cetuximab, with radiotherapy also increases survival, without a significant increase in toxicity. These results offer the possibility of introducing this new treatment combination into more routine practice, and also the possibility of exploring the effect of combining cetuximab with cisplatin-based chemoradiation. Trials are also underway with VEGFR inhibitor bevacizumab, in combination with radiotherapy.

Giving conventional adjuvant cytotoxic chemotherapy after surgery or radiotherapy has not been shown to clearly improve long-term survival. However, the observation that when patients relapse after chemoradiation it is usually because of distant metastases, rather than local recurrence of the disease, has led to the suggestion that induction, or neoadjuvant, chemotherapy, given prior to the chemoradiation might improve the long-term results. Clinical trials using combinations of either paclitaxel or docetaxel with cisplatin and fluorouracil as induction therapies have shown promising results. For patients with locally advanced, bulky disease, neoadjuvant therapy also acts as a good predictor of response to radiotherapy, with patients achieving a good partial response being likely to benefit from intensive chemoradiation whereas those who show no obvious tumour shrinkage are unlikely to benefit from this intensive regimen and should probably be offered the gentler option of radiotherapy alone.

For patients who do relapse with local recurrence then salvage surgical measures with either conventional resections or laser surgery may be helpful. As far as chemotherapy is concerned cytotoxic treatment is of limited value but the combination of cisplatin and fluorouracil is often used. For those patients who achieve a good response and go on to relapse more than 3 months after completion of their treatment, second-line therapy with cytotoxics such as methotrexate or one of the taxanes may be worth a try.

Suggestions for further reading

Bonner JA, Harari PM, Giralt J et al. Radiotherapy plus cetuximab for squamous cell carcinoma of the head and neck. N Engl J Med, 2006; 354: 567–578.

Hwang D, O'Sullivan B. What's new in the non-surgical treatment of head and neck cancer? Oncology News, 2007; 1: 12–14.

James N, Hartley A. Improving outcomes in head and neck cancer. Clin Oncol, 2003; 15: 264–265.

Seiwert TY, Cohen EEW. State-of-the-art management of locally advanced head and neck cancer. Br J Cancer, 2005; 92: 1341–1348.

SKIN CANCER

The principal types of skin cancer are basal cell carcinomas, squamous cell carcinomas and malignant melanoma. The great majority of skin cancers in the UK are either basal or squamous cell carcinomas, with more than 100,000 cases being diagnosed each year. Chemotherapy plays virtually no part in the management of these cancers, but occasionally topical application of fluorouracil cream (in concentrations of 0.5%–5%) may be recommended for very superficial basal cell carcinomas.

Each year there are about 8,000 new cases of malignant melanoma, making it the eighth commonest cancer in the UK.

There are 1,800 deaths annually from malignant melanoma in UK. The first-line management of localized melanoma is surgery, with a wide local excision. The 5-year survival rate for men is about 80% and for women it is about 90%.

Numerous clinical trials have explored the role of adjuvant chemotherapy for the more advanced stages of localized disease, but none has yet shown a convincing benefit. For patients who are keen to explore adjuvant therapy the recommendation should be for them to enter an appropriate clinical trial.

Metastatic melanoma is a relatively chemoresistant disease. The drug which has been most extensively explored in this indication is the cytotoxic dacarbazine (DTIC). Used as a single agent this has produced partial response rates ranging from 15% to 30%, and complete responses in 3%–5% of patients; however there is no convincing evidence that treatment leads to any increase in survival. Similarly although some trials combining DTIC with other cytotoxics, or interferon, have claimed higher response rates, there are still no clear data to support the view that life-expectancy is prolonged, compared to giving best supportive care.

Suggestions for further reading

ESMO. Minimum clinical recommendations for diagnosis, treatment and follow-up of cutaneous malignant melanoma. Annals Oncol, 2005; 16 (supplement 1): i66–i68.

Thompson JF, Scolyer RA, Kefford RF. Cutaneous melanoma. Lancet, 2005; 365: 687–701.

Tsao H, Atkins MB, Sober AJ. Management of cutaneous melanoma. New Engl J Med, 2004; 351: 998–1012.

Wong CSM, Strange RC, Lear JT. Basal cell carcinoma. Br Med J, 2003; 327: 794–798.

SOFT-TISSUE SARCOMAS

There are about 2,200 new cases of soft-tissue sarcoma each year in UK, making up about 1% of all cancers. Just under 1,000 people die annually of the disease. The average age at the time of diagnosis is the early 60s, although these tumours may occur at any age. Soft-tissue sarcomas make up a very diverse group of cancers (Table 3.1). Of these growths 50% occur in the limbs, 40% in the trunk or retroperitoneum and 10% in the head and neck. The overall 5-year survival figure in the UK is between 50% and 60%, although the figures do vary considerably for different tumour types and sites; for example, retroperitoneal soft-tissue sarcomas tend to have a poorer outlook, largely because of their

TABLE 3.1. Relative incidence of soft-tissue sarcoma*

	All sites	Soft tissues only
Leiomyosarcoma	24%	12%
Malignant fibrous histiocytoma	17%	25%
Liposarcoma	12%	24%
Dermatofibrosarcoma	11%	2%
Rhabdomysarcoma	5%	5%
Angiosarcoma	4%	4%
Nerve sheath tumours	4%	6%
Fibrosarcoma	4%	5%

* Soft-tissue sarcomas may occur either in specific organs or in the soft tissues, and the incidence of the different types of sarcoma differs between the two sites. Approximately 50% of the sarcomas occur in soft tissues and 50% in specific organs. Among the latter the commonest are skin (28%), uterus (14%), the retroperitoneum (14%), stomach (8%) and small intestine (6%).

later presentation. The size and histological grade of the sarcoma are also important prognostic features with larger tumours, >5cm, and high grade, grade III, cancers (which account for about 50% of these growths), faring worse.

Wherever possible surgery is the treatment of choice for these lesions, with removal of the primary cancer, and a margin of at least 2cm of surrounding normal tissue. When there is doubt about the completeness of the excision, or for larger, high-grade lesions, then post-operative radiotherapy is usually recommended.

Results suggest that adjuvant chemotherapy is of limited value. Local and distant relapse may be delayed by treatment but there are no convincing data that overall survival is increased. Clinical trials in this area are still continuing, particularly for larger lesions. Neoadjuvant, pre-operative chemotherapy is sometimes used for larger sarcomas, to try and improve the surgical outcome.

Soft-tissue sarcomas tend to spread predominately to the lungs, and resection of isolated lung metastases may sometimes be a treatment option in advanced disease. Cytotoxic chemotherapy is of only limited value. The most active agents are doxorubicin and ifosfamide. When used as single agents they have a response rate of about 20%. Given in combination with dacarbazine, this figure rises to between 30% and 35%, but this is quite an aggressive regimen, most suitable for younger fitter patients.

One type of soft-tissue sarcoma that merits special mention is gastrointestinal stromal tumour (GIST). These have been distinguished as a separate entity in the last decade, many previously being considered leiomyosarcomas These are the commonest sarcoma of the gastrointestinal tract, with about 800 new cases in UK each year. Surgery is the primary treatment wherever possible. Conventional cytotoxics are ineffective for more advanced stages of the disease, but more than 80% of these cancers carry a KIT gene mutation and are susceptible to the tyrosine kinase inhibitor imatinib. As a result these patients with advanced disease will gain a response lasting in excess of 2 years on average, and their median 5-year survival will be about 5 years, compared with only 1 year before imatinib was introduced. Another tyrosine kinase inhibitor, sunitinib, is currently being evaluated for use in patients with relapsed or resistant GIST following imatinib therapy.

Suggestions for further reading

Clark MA, Fisher C, Judson I, Thomas JM. Soft-tissue sarcomas in adults. New Engl J Med, 2005; 353: 701–711.

Joensuu H. Sunitinib for imatinib-resistant GIST. Lancet, 2006; 368: 1303–1304.

ESMO. Minimum clinical recommendations for diagnosis, treatment and follow-up of soft tissue sarcomas. Annals Oncol, 2005; 16 (supplement 1): i69–i70.

Toro JR, Travis LB, Wu HJ et al. Incidence patterns of soft tissue sarcoma, regardless of primary site, in the surveillance, epidemiology and end results program, 1978–2001: an analysis of 26,758 cases. Int J Cancer, 2006; 119: 2922–2930.

Verweij J, Casali PG, Zalcberg J et al. Progression-free survival in gastrointestinal stromal tumours with high-dose imatinib: randomized trial. Lancet, 2004; 364: 1127–1134.

PRIMARY BONE SARCOMAS

There are about 450 new cases of bone sarcomas each year in UK, making up about 0.2% of all cancers. About 200 people die annually of the disease. The majority of these cancers occur between the ages of 10 and 20, although there is a second peak in the over 60s which accounts for about 10% of cases. Primary bone tumours are common in men than women with a ratio of 3:2. The overall 5-year survival figure in the UK is just over 50%. Osteosarcomas are the commonest type of primary bone sarcoma, other types are Ewing's sarcoma, chondrosarcoma and spindle cell sarcomas (the latter being made up of a variety of tumour types, generally behaving in a similar way to osteosarcoma, and occurring in older people).

For osteosarcomas treatment is based on a combination of surgery and chemotherapy. Surgery is aimed at removing the primary tumour, which may involve an amputation. Cytotoxic chemotherapy is given pre-operatively (neoadjuvant therapy), to shrink the primary lesion, facilitating surgery, and is continued as post-operative adjuvant therapy. The most widely used treatment schedule is based on giving cisplatin and doxorubicin (on days 1 and 2) on a 5-week cycle and high-dose methorexate (on days 22 and 29) followed by leucovorin rescue. This is an aggressive regimen with a high incidence of toxicity. Other drugs which may be used in these tumours include cyclophospahmide, ifosfamide and etoposide.

For Ewing's sarcoma radiotherapy or surgery is used to treat the primary growth but adjuvant cytotoxic chemotherapy is then essential to maximize the chance of cure. In the UK and Europe favoured treatment schedules are vincristine, ifosfamide, doxorubicin and etoposide (VIDE) given every 3 weeks for 6 courses, or vincristine, ifosfamide and dactinomycin (VIA) given every 3 weeks for 8 courses. In North America combinations of either vincristine, doxorubicin and cyclophosphamide or ifosfamide and etoposide tend to be preferred.

Treatment of chondrosarcomas and spindle cell sarcomas tends to be similar to that of osteosarcoma, although the chemotherapy schedules may be less intense as it is generally an older group of patients who are being treated.

Suggestions for further reading

ESMO. Minimum clinical recommendations for diagnosis, treatment and follow-up of osteosarcoma. Annals Oncol, 2005; 16 (supplement 1): i71–i72.

ESMO. Minimum clinical recommendations for diagnosis, treatment and follow-up of Ewing's sarcoma of bone. Annals Oncol, 2005; 16 (supplement 1): i73–i74.

HAEMATOLOGICAL CANCER

Acute Lymphoblastic Leukaemia

Acute lymphoblastic leukaemia (ALL) is a disease of progenitor cells of either B-cell or T-cell lymphocytes. In ALL these cells escape from normal growth control mechanisms and lose the ability to differentiate, remaining as primitive blast cells, appearing in the peripheral blood and infiltrating the bone marrow.

There are about 550 new cases of ALL each year in UK. Of these about two-thirds are in children and adolescents, with a peak age of 3–4 years. In adults the median age at diagnosis ranges from 25 to 37, this reflects a high incidence in young adults, and a second peak occurring in those over 75.

Progressive improvements in chemotherapy and supportive care over the last 50 years mean that in children the overall cure rate is in excess of 80%. Unfortunately the figure is far worse in adults, being about 40%. Age is a strong prognostic factor in adults, with older people faring worse. About 25% of adults, and 5% of children, with ALL will have leukaemic cells which carry the Philadelphia chromosome (see Section 'Chronic Myeloid Leukaemia').

In both adults and children there are four components to treatment: remission induction, consolidation or intensification, maintenance and CNS prophylaxis.

For children remission induction typically involves the use of a steroid (either prednisone, prednisolone, or dexamethasone), vincristine and asparaginase. For those with a poor prognosis, and most young adults, an anthracycline, usually daunorubicin will be added. For those adults with the Philadelphia chromosome the tyrosine kinase inhibitor, imatinib is added to their drug regimen. Treatment extends over 4–6 weeks, with the aim of destroying 99% or more of the leukaemic cells. The treatment is intensive and requires rigorous supportive care with red cell and platelet transfusions and infection prophylaxis, so it is done on an in-patient basis. The response to remission induction is a strong prognostic marker, with those who fail to gain a complete remission within 4 weeks having a poor outlook.

For those who achieve a remission the next stage is intensification, or consolidation. This involves a variety of different regimens depending on the patient's age and the precise subtype of ALL. Typical treatments include high-dose methorexate with mercaptopurine, or high-dose asparaginase or a repeat of the original induction regimen. This phase usually lasts for 4–8 weeks. An alternative at this stage, particularly for young adults, is an allogeneic stem-cell transplant.

Maintenance or continuation therapy involves gentler, long-term chemotherapy, for between 2 and 3 years. The most widely used combination is daily oral mercaptopurine with weekly oral methotrexate. Adults with the Philadelphia chromosome will also continue imatinib.

Unless treatment is given, between 30% and 50% of people who achieve a remission will relapse with CNS involvement by their leukaemia. It is impossible to predict who will develop this problem so treatment known as 'CNS prophylaxis' is almost universally given. This used to involve radiotherapy to the brain and spinal cord, but this led to the risk of long-term complications of a degree of mental impairment and pituitary damage, so is now generally avoided. The usual alternative is intrathecal administration of methotrexate. Depending on individual treatment protocols, this may be given as part of remission induction, or intensification, or maintenance or at all three stages of treatment.

Suggestion for further reading
Pui C-H, Evans WE. Treatment of acute lymphoblastic leukemia. N Engl J Med 2006; 354: 166–178.

Acute Myeloid Leukaemia
Acute myeloid leukaemia (AML) is a disease of bone marrow stem cells, which produce red blood cells, neutrophils and platelets. In AML these cells escape from normal growth control mechanisms and lose the ability to differentiate, remaining as primitive blast cells. When the bone marrow contains more than 20% of blast cells then AML is diagnosed. Failure of red cell and platelet formation lead to anaemia and bleeding disorders and the absence of mature neutrophils leads to infection, which is the usual cause of death.

There are about 2,000 new cases of AML each year in UK, with an average age at diagnosis of 70. There are a number of different types of AML and 55% of people with the disease show specific cytogenetic abnormalities in their blast cells which allow not only for precise classification of their AML subtype but also give a guide to prognosis. Age is a major prognostic factor, with people over 55–60 faring far worse than younger adults. Performance status and a number of biochemical measures, such as serum albumin, bilirubin and creatinine levels, also influence outcome.

For younger adults, below the age of 60, the cornerstone of treatment is induction of complete remission which typically relies on a regimen of the cytotoxics daunorubicin (given iv on 3 consecutive days) and cytarabine (given by continuous iv infusion for 7–10 days). This combination will produce a complete remission (defined as <5% blasts in the bone marrow) in 65–75% of people. Other drugs which may be used in remission induction are etoposide, fludarabine and idarubicin. Clinical trials are also in progress assessing whether adding gemtuzumab will improve the outcome. Gemtuzumab is a conjugate of a monoclonal antibody, which targets the CD33 protein on the leukaemic cells, and a cytotoxic called calicheamicin. In one specific type of AML – acute promyelocytic leukaemia – the drug ALL trans-retinoic acid, derived from vitamin A, is highly effective and is combined with an anthracycline cytotoxic in remission induction.

Once a remission has been achieved the next stage is consolidation therapy, which for good and intermediate prognosis individuals involves one of a number of regimens. Among the commonest of these are high-dose cytarabine therapy or a repeat of two courses of induction therapy, followed by a course of amsacrine, cytarabine and etoposide followed by a final course of mitoxantrone and cytarabine. Once again ALL-trans-retinoic acid is of value in acute promyelocytic leukaemia. Unlike acute lymphoblastic leukaemia there is no benefit in giving long-term maintenance therapy, or CNS Prophylaxis. For the poor risk group options include allogeneic stem cell transplants or experimental therapies. Depending on prognostic factors, the overall cure rate for this age group lies between 20% and 75%.

For older patients options include standard daunorubicin–cytarabine, experimental therapy and supportive care. Overall, however, the outcomes are disappointing with less than 10% of people being cured, and the average survival only stretching to 10 months.

Suggestions for further reading

British Committee for Standards in Haematology. Guidelines on the management of acute myeloid leukaemia in adults. Br J Haemtol 2006; 135: 450–474.

ESMO. Minimum clinical recommendations for diagnosis, treatment and follow-up of acute myeloblastic leukemia (AML). Annals Oncol, 2005; 16 (supplement 1): i48–i49.

Estey E, Dohner H. Acute myeloid leukaemia. Lancet 2006; 368: 1894–1907.

Chronic Myeloid Leukaemia

As with acute myeloid leukaemia the underlying abnormality is overproduction of bone marrow stem cells. Of the people with chronic myeloid leukaemia (CML), 95% have a translocation between chromosomes 9 and 22, producing what is known as the Philadelphia chromosome. This translocation produces a fusion gene, *brc-abl*, which in turn generates a specific tyrosine kinase pathway which stimulates cell division.

There are about 650 new cases of CML in UK each year, with 66 as an average age of onset(although about 2% of cases occur in children). The disease goes through three phases. Firstly there is the chronic phase, which lasts about 3–5 years. Often a raised white cell count is the only abnormality during this time and symptoms are few, the condition frequently being diagnosed as the result of a routine blood test. This is followed by the accelerated phase which lasts anywhere from 2 to 15 months. During this time anaemia and splenomegaly develop causing symptoms of tiredness and abdominal discomfort, and an increased risk of infection and bleeding problems. Finally there is the blast crisis which lasts just a few months. This is essentially a transformation to an acute myeloid leukaemia and is invariably fatal.

An allogeneic stem cell transplant is the only curative option for CML but most patients are too old for this to be considered. In recent years the drug treatment of CML has been transformed by the discovery of imatinib. This is a signal transduction inhibitor which specifically blocks *brc-abl* tyrosine kinase activity. When given to people in the chronic phase of CML more than 95% gain a response with nearly 90% still being alive after 5 years. Treatment with imatinib is continued indefinitely as even complete responders appear to be at risk of relapse if the drug is stopped.

Treatment options for people who relapse on imatinib include interferon, cytotoxic chemotherapy with drugs like hydroxyurea, busulphan, or cytarabine, or an allogeneic stem cell transplant, but the outcomes are uncertain. However, early trials with two new *brc-abl* tyrosine kinase inhibitors called dasatinib and nilotinib indicate that they might be effective in overcoming resistance to imatinib and may offer another therapeutic option in the future.

Suggestion for further reading
Druker BJ, Guilhot F, O'Brien SG et al. Five-year follow-up of patients receiving imatinib for chronic myeloid leukaemia. N Engl J Med 2006; 355: 2408–2417.

ESMO. Minimum clinical recommendations for diagnosis, treatment and follow-up of chronic myelogenous leukemia. Annals Oncol, 2005; 16 (supplement 1): i52–i53.

Chronic Lymphocytic Leukaemia

In chronic lymphocytic leukaemia (CLL) the underlying abnormality is an overproduction of lymphocytes, which appear in the bone marrow, the circulating blood and lymph node masses. Rather confusingly CLL is also classified as a form of low-grade, non-Hodgkin's lymphoma (NHL).

There are about 4,500 new cases of CLL each year in UK. The average age of onset is between 65 and 70. The overall median life-expectancy from the time of diagnosis is around 10 years, but there are wide individual variations. Between 75% and 80% of cases are asymptomatic and discovered as the result of routine blood tests, in the remainder the presenting symptoms are usually either enlarged lymph nodes or tiredness due to anaemia.

The disease is normally indolent, and asymptomatic patients often require no treatment initially. Indications for starting therapy include progressive bone marrow failure (with either anaemia or thrombocytopenia), enlarging lymph nodes or progressive splenomegaly, a rapid increase in the number of circulating lymphocytes, or the onset of systemic symptoms such as weight loss or fever.

In contrast to CML there is no good evidence that treatment during the indolent phase of the disease improves the outcome. First-line active treatment is based on cytotoxic chemotherapy with the main choices being either chlorambucil or fludarabine. Both these agents can be given orally and result in remissions in 75%–80% of patients, with about 30%–40% of these being complete remissions, median survival at 5 years about 50%. On relapse further responses can often be obtained by either rechallenging with the original drug or changing from one to the other. Alternatively intravenous infusions of cyclohposhamide or cladribine may be used. For more resistant disease combined cytotoxic treatment can be tried, with cyclophosphamide and fludarabine, or cyclophosphamide, vincristine and prednisolone, or cyclophoshamide doxorubicin and prednisolone. Monoclonal antibodies may also be used, giving either alemtuzumab alone or rituximab in combination with fludarabine and cyclophosphamide. For younger patients an allogeneic transplant is an option and offers the only chance of cure, although the procedure is not without its risks and carries a mortality of about 20%. The enlarged lymph node masses which occur are very sensitive to radiotherapy and this may also be used to help control the disease in its more advanced stages. High-dose steroid therapy may also be useful at this time.

Suggestion for further reading

British Committee for Standards in Haematology. Guidelines on the diagnosis and management of chronic lymphocytic leukaemia. Br J Haemtol 2004; 125: 294–317.

ESMO. Minimum clinical recommendations for diagnosis, treatment and follow-up of chronic lymphocytic leukemia. Annals Oncol, 2005; 16 (supplement 1): i50–i51.

Lymphomas

Lymphomas are traditionally divided into Hodgkin's lymphoma and non-Hodgkin's lymphoma. Hodgkin's lymphoma is named after the English physician, Thomas Hodgkin, who first described the disease in the 1880s, and is distinguished from the other lymphoma by the presence of a specific type of abnormal B-lymphocyte: the Reed-Sternberg cell.

Hodgkin's Lymphoma

There are about 1,400 new cases of Hodgkin's lymphoma each year in UK. The peak age of incidence is in young adults, between 16–15, although people of any age may be affected. Discovery of a swollen lymph node mass is the usual presenting feature but occasionally systemic symptoms, such as weight loss, fever, to generalized itching, may dominate the picture. Forty years ago the condition was almost universally fatal but as a result firstly of wide-field radiotherapy and then of developments in combination chemotherapy the overall cure rate is now in excess of 75%.

The choice of treatment depends on the specific cellular sub-type of Hodgkin's lymphoma (Table 3.2), the stage of the disease (Table 3.3) and other prognostic factors. From these, four subgroups can be identified.

1. *Early favourable disease: non-bulky stage IA or II A.* These patients used to be treated by wide-field radiotherapy, but concerns about the risk of second malignancies and other long-term complications have led to an increasing preference for cytotoxic chemotherapy. Drug regimens that have been used include MOPP (nitrogen mustard, vincristine, procarbazine and prednisone), BEACOPP (bleomycin, etoposide, doxorubicin, cyclophosphamide, vincristine, procarbazine and prednisone) and ABVD (doxorubicin, bleomycin, vinblastine and dacarbazine). Although MOPP was the pioneer combination which revolutionized the outcome in Hodgkin's lymphoma, both MOPP and BEACOPP almost always lead to infertility and also carry about a 3% risk of developing

TABLE 3.2. Hodgkin's lymphoma: Cellular classification

Classical Hodgkin's lymphoma
    Nodular sclerosis
    Mixed-cellularity
    Lymphocyte depleted
    Lymphocyte-rich classical
Nodular lymphocyte-predominant HL
    This is a more indolent form of the disease, with a tendency to recur.

TABLE 3.3. The staging of Hodgkin's lymphoma (simplified)

I Involvement of a single lymph node region
II Involvement of two or more lymph node regions on the same side of the diaphragm
III Involvement of lymph node regions on both sides of the diaphragm
IV Multifocal involvement of one or more extralymphatic organs

These stages may be subclassified as A or B. The B designation is given to people with one or more of the following symptoms:

- unexplained weight loss of more than 10%
- unexplained fever with temperatures above 38°C
- drenching night sweats

secondary acute leukaemia. By contrast ABVD has little effect on fertility and has <1% risk of leukaemia, so has become the preferred treatment. For these patients the treatment options are either 4–6 courses of ABVD or 4 courses of ABVD followed by radiotherapy to the involved lymph node sites or, if disease was very localized, radiotherapy alone to the involved lymph nodes. These will result in a cure rate in excess of 90%.

2. *Early unfavourable disease: stage IA or IIA with B symptoms, bulky disease or other adverse prognostic factors*. Bulky disease is defined as lymph node masses greater than 10cm in diameter, or mediastinal disease greater than one-third of the thoracic diameter. The usual choice of treatment here is either 4–6 cycles of ABVD or 4 cycles of ABVD followed by radiotherapy to the involved lymph node sites. This will result in a cure rate in excess of 80%.

3. *Advanced favourable disease: stage III or IV disease with few adverse prognostic factors*. The most widely used regimen is 6–8 cycles of ABVD, which may be followed by local radiotherapy if there was bulky disease. This will result in a cure rate of about 60%.

4. *Advanced unfavourable disease: stage III or IV with poor prognostic factors*. Options here include either 6–8 cycles of ABVD or 6–8 cycles of BEACOPP. These will give a cure rate of up to 50%.

Non-Hodgkin's Lymphoma

These are a diverse group of cancers and over the last 30 years more than 25 different systems have been suggested for their classification. Currently the most widely accepted system is the REAL/WHO classification. From a clinical viewpoint these various conditions can be grouped into indolent, or low-grade

TABLE 3.4. Principal types of non-Hodgkin's lymphoma, and their incidence

Low grade	
B-cell cancers	
Follicular lymphoma	22%
Extranodal marginal zone	
lymphoma (MALT lymphoma)	8%
B-cell small lymphocytic lymphoma/	
chronic lymphocytic leukaemia	7%
Nodal marginal zone lymphoma	2%
Lymphoplasmacytic lymphoma/	
Waldentrom's macroglobulinaemia	1%
High grade	
B-cell cancers	
Diffuse large B-cell lymphoma	33%
Mantle cell lymphoma	6%
Burkitt's lymphoma	2%
T-cell cancers	
Mature (peripheral) T-cell neoplasms	8%
Precursor T-lymphoblastic lymphoma/leukaemia	
	2%
Primary systemic anaplastic large cell lymphoma	
	2%

NHL, or aggressive or high-grade NHL (Table 3.4). Overall survival at 5 years is about 50%–60%.

There are about 5,500 new cases of low-grade NHL and 2,200 of high-grade NHL, each year in UK, and the incidence of the disease is steadily increasing at a rate of about 3% per year. Overall NHL is the sixth commonest cancer in the UK. Although the average age of onset is 55–60, people of any age may be affected. The clinical presentations vary widely but the discovery of enlarged lymph node masses is the most common. The staging system for NHL is similar to that of Hodgkin's lymphoma, although most people present with stage III or IV disease.

Although treatment varies with the individual type of NHL, the broad principles of managing low-grade and high-grade disease are as follows.

Low-grade disease: In a few instances the disease will be truly localized, confined to one or two groups of lymph nodes, and in this situation radiotherapy may result in a cure. In all other situations low-grade NHL is usually incurable, although the disease often progresses very slowly, with an overall median survival of about 10 years. Because of its slow progression and relative lack of symptoms, some people may need no immediate treatment and can enter a policy of watchful waiting, being regularly monitored with treatment being reserved until there are clear signs of disease progression. When treatment is needed cytotoxic chemotherapy is the usual choice, and options include oral chlorambucil as a single agent, or combination regimens with either CVP (cyclophosphamide, vincristine and prednisone) or CHOP (cyclophosphamide, doxorubicin, vincristine and prednisone). In recent years there is evidence that adding a monoclonal antibody, rituximab, to CVP or CHOP may enhance the duration of remissions. Rituximab binds to a protein called CD20 which is found on the surface of normal and malignant B-cell lymphocytes. Malignant B-cell lymphocytes are the dominant cancer cell type in most types of low-grade NHL. Although these drugs will bring about complete remissions for many people, the disease will ultimately recur and re-treatment will be necessary.

High-grade NHL: Paradoxically, although it is more aggressive, the chances of cure are greater with high-grade than low-grade NHL, with between 30–60% of people surviving long term. Chemotherapy is the cornerstone of treatment with either CHOP or R-CHOP (CHOP + rituximab) for 4–8 courses. For some patients this may be followed by radiotherapy to the involved lymph node areas. For some younger patients, who have gone into remission but who are considered to be at high risk of relapse, bone marrow or stem cell transplantation may be considered.

Suggestions for further reading

Bonadonna G, Viviani S, Bonfante V et al. Survival in Hodgkin's disease patients–report of 25 years of experience at the Milan Cancer Institute. Eur J Cancer 2005; 41: 998–1006.

ESMO. Minimum clinical recommendations for diagnosis, treatment and follow-up of Hodgkin's disease. Annals Oncol, 2005; 16 (supplement 1): i54–i55.

ESMO. Minimum clinical recommendations for diagnosis, treatment and follow-up of newly diagnosed follicular lymphoma. Annals Oncol, 2005; 16 (supplement 1): i56–i57.

ESMO. Minimum clinical recommendations for diagnosis, treatment and follow-up of newly diagnosed large cell non-Hodgkin's lymphoma. Annals Oncol, 2005; 16 (supplement 1): i58–i59.

ESMO. Minimum clinical recommendations for diagnosis, treatment and follow-up of relapsed large cell non-Hodgkin's lymphoma. Annals Oncol, 2005; 16 (supplement 1): i60–i61.

Evans LS, Hancock BW. Non-Hodgkin's lymphoma. Lancet 2003; 362: 139–146.

Multiple Myeloma

The underlying abnormality in multiple myeloma is a proliferation of abnormal plasma cells (plasma cells are derived from B-lymphocytes and are responsible for antibody production). These settle in the bone marrow and cause destruction of the surrounding bone, leading to pain and fractures. Normal plasma cells are involved in antibody formation and produce immunoglobulins, their malignant counterparts usually produce abnormal amounts of specific immunoglobulins and the high concentrations of these can lead to complications such as renal failure.

There are about 3,300 new cases of multiple myeloma each year in UK. The median age at presentation is about 70, and fewer than 2% of patients are diagnosed under 40. Bone pain is the commonest presenting symptom. The condition is incurable but survival times are very variable, ranging from a few months to more than 20 years.

Some people may be asymptomatic when multiple myeloma is first diagnosed, and for them it is often safe to withhold treatment until there is evidence of disease progression, which may be anywhere from 1 to 3 years. Once treatment is indicated the choice of therapy is determined by a number of factors, including the patient's age and general fitness. For younger patients, below the ages of 55–65, some form of high-dose chemotherapy and bone marrow or stem cell transplant may be considered. In this situation the first-line treatment is likely to be cytotoxic therapy with either VAD (vincristine, doxorubicin and dexamethasone), VAMP (vincristine, doxorubicin, methorexate and prednisone) or C-VAMP (VAMP + cyclophosphamide). For the majority of people, however, a gentler oral treatment will usually be indicated with either melphalan or cyclophosphamide, plus or minus prednisone. This is usually continued for up to 3 months following the achievement of a maximal response.

Two new agents which are showing promise in multiple myeloma are thalidomide, which is an anti-angionenic agent, and bortezomib, which is a proteasome inhibitor. At present these drugs are mainly used as second- or third-line therapies, following a relapse, but a number of trials are assessing their value in the earlier stages of treatment.

Bone pain is a major problem in multiple myeloma. Successful chemotherapy often eases the problem but for those people where symptoms persist localized radiotherapy (usually only requiring a single low-dose treatment) or bisphosphonates given orally or by 4–6 weekly iv infusions may be very beneficial. Bisphosphonates also help reduce the risk of bone fractures and spinal cord compression.

Suggestions for further reading

ESMO. Minimum clinical recommendations for diagnosis, treatment and follow-up of multiple myeloma. Annals Oncol, 2005; 16 (supplement 1): i45–i47.

NICE. NICE appraisal of bortezomib for the treatment of relapsed and refractory multiple myeloma. October 2006. www.nice.org.uk

Siroki B, Powles R. Multiple myeloma. Lancet 2004; 363: 875–887.

Smith A, Wisloff F, Samson D. Guidelines on the diagnosis and management of multiple myeloma 2005. Br J Haematol 2005; 132: 410–451.

Appendix I
Chemotherapeutic Agents and Their Trade Names in the UK

Alkylating agents
Busulfan (Myleran, Busilvex)
Carmustine, BCNU (BiCNU, Gliadel wafers)
Chlorambucil (Leukeran)
Cyclophosphamide (Endoxana)
Dacarbazine, DTIC
Ifosfamide (Mitoxana)
Lomustine, CCNU (Lomustine)

Melphalan (Alkeran)
Mitomycin (Mitomycin C Kyowa)

Nitrogen mustard
Procarbazine
Temozolamide (Temodal)
Thiotepa
Treosulfan (Tresosulfan)

Platinum analogues
Carboplatin (Paraplatin)
Cisplatin

Oxaliplatin (Eloxatin)

Antimetabolites
Captecitabine (Xeloda)
Cladribine (Leustat, Litak)
Cytaribine (lipid formulation: DepoCyte)
Fludarabine (Fludara)
Fluorouracil (topical: Efudix)
Gemcitabine (Gemzar)
Hydroxyurea (Hydrea)

Mercaptopurine (Puri-nethol)
Methotrexate
Pemetrexed (Alimta)

Pentostatin (Nipent)
Raltitrexed (Tomudex)
Tegafur with uracil (Uftoral)
Thioguanine, tioguanine (Lanvis)

Topoisomerase I inhibitors
Irinotecan (Campto)

Topotecan (Hycamtin)

Topoisomerase II inhibitors
Amsacrine (Amisidine)
Daunorubicin (lipid formulation: DaunoXome)
Doxorubicin (Adriamycin, lipid Formulation: Caelyx, Myocet)
Epirubicin (Pharmorubicin)

Etoposide (Etophos, Vepesid)
Idarubicin (Zavedos)

Mitoxantrone (Onkotrone, Mitoxantrone)

continued

Cytotoxic antibiotics
Bleomycin (Bleomyicn)

Dactinomycin, actinomycin D (Cosmogen Lyovac)

Anti-microtubule drugs
Docetaxel (Taxotere)
Paclitaxel (Placlitaxel, Taxol)
Vinblastine (Velbe)

Vincristine (Oncovin)
Vindesine (Eldisine)
Vinorelbine (Navelbine)

Targeted therapies
Alemtuzumab (MabCampath)
Bevacizumab (Avastin)
Bortezomib (Velcade)
Cetuximab (Erbitux)
Erlotinib (Tarceva)
Gefitinib (Iressa)
Imatinib (Glivec)

Lapatinib (Tykerb)
Nilotinib (AMN 107)
Rituximab (MabThera)
Sorafinib (Nexavar)
Sunitinib (Sutent)
Temsirolimus CCI779
Trastuzumab (Herceptin)

Cytokines
Interferon alpha (IntronA, Roferon-A, Viraferon)

Interleukin, aldesleukin (Proleukin)

Sex hormones and hormone antagonists
Anastrazole (Arimidex)
Bicalutamide (Casodex)
Buserilin (Suprefact)

Cyproterone acetate (Cyprostat)
Exemestane (Aromasin)
Flutamide (Drogenil)
Fulvestrant (Faslodex)
Goserelin (Zoladex)

Letrozole (Femara)
Leuprorelin (Prostap)
Medroxyprogesterone (Farlutal, Provera)
Megestrol acetate (Megace)
Norethisterone
Stilboestrol (Diethylstilboestrol)
Tamoxifen (Nolvadex-D)
Triptorelin (Decapeptyl, Gonapeptyl)

Where no brand name is given, none currently exists in the UK

Appendix 2

Acronyms of Some Commonly Used Chemotherapy Regimens

Acronym	Drugs used	Indication(s)
ABVD	doxorubicin (**A**driamycin), **b**leomycin, **v**inblastine, **d**acarbazine	Hodgkin's lymphoma
AC	doxorubicin (**A**driamycin), **c**yclophosphamide	Breast cancer
ACE cancer	doxorubicin (**A**driamycin), **c**yclophosphamide, **e**toposide	Small-cell lung
AT	doxorubicin (**A**driamycin), docetaxel (**T**axotere)	Breast cancer
BEP	**b**leomycin, **e**toposide, **c**isplatin	Testicular cancer, dysgerminoma ovary
C-VAMP	**c**yclophosphamide, **v**incristine, doxorubicin (**A**driamycin), **m**ethyl-**p**rednisolone	Multiple myeloma
CAF	**c**yclophosphamide, doxorubicin (**A**driamycin), **f**luorouracil	Breast cancer
CarboMV	**carbo**platin, **m**ethotrexate, **v**inlbastine	Bladder cancer
CAV	**c**yclophosphamide, doxorubicin (**A**driamycin), **v**incristine	Small cell lung cancer
ChlVPP	**chl**orambucil, **v**inblastine, **p**rocarbazine, **p**rednisolone	Hodgkin's lymphoma
CHOP	**c**yclophosphamide, doxorubicin (doxorubicin **h**ydrochloride), vincristine (**O**ncovin), **p**rednisolone	Non-Hodgkin's lymphoma
CMF	cyclophosphamide, **m**ethorexate, **f**luorouracil	Breast cancer

continued

Acronym	Drugs used	Indication(s)
CYVADIC	**cy**clophosphamide, **v**incristine, doxorubicin (**Ad**riamycin), dacarbazine (DT**IC**)	Soft-tissue sarcoma
de Gramont	leucovorin, bolus fluorouracil, 22 hour infusion fluorouracil on days 1 & 2, every 14 days	Colorectal cancer
DHAP	**d**examet**h**asone, cytarabine (cytosine **a**rabinoside), cis**p**latin	Non-Hodgkin's lymphoma
E-CMF	**e**pirubicin, **c**yclophosphamide, **m**ehotrexate, **f**luorouracil	Breast cancer
EC	**e**pirubicin, **c**yclophosphamide	Breast cancer
EC	**e**toposide, **c**isplatin	Small cell lung cancer
ECF	**e**pirubicin, **c**isplatin, **f**luorouracil	Stomach, esophageal and ovarian cancer
ECX	**e**pirubicin, **c**isplatin, capecitabine (**X**eloda)	Stomach, esophageal cancer
EEX	**e**pirubicin, oxaliplatin (**E**loxatin), capecitabine (**X**eloda)	Stomach, esophageal cancer
ELF	**e**toposide, **l**eucovorin, **f**luorouracil	Stomach, esophageal cancer
FAM	**f**luorouracil, doxorubicin (**A**driamycin), **M**itomycin	Stomach, pancreatic cancer
FEC	**f**luorouracil, **e**pirubicin, **c**yclophosphamide	Breast cancer
Gemcap	**g**emcitabine, **c**apecitabine	Pancreatic cancer
Gemcarbo	**g**emcitabine, **c**arboplatin	Small cell and non-small-cell lung cancer
Gemcis	**g**emcitabine, **c**isplatin	Pancreatic and non-small cell lung cancer
ICE	**i**fosfamide, **c**arboplatin, **e**toposide cancer	Small-cell lung Non-Hodgkin's lymphoma
MACOP-B	**m**ethotrexate, doxorubicin (**A**driamycin), **c**yclophosphamide, vincristine (**O**ncovin), **p**rednisolone, **b**leomycin	Non-Hodgkin's lymphoma

continued

Acronym	Drugs used	Indication(s)
Mayo	bolus fluorouracil and leucovorin daily for five days once every four weeks	Colorectal cancer
MIC	**m**itomycin, **i**fosfamide, **c**isplatin	Non-small cell lung cancer
MM	**m**ethotrexate, **m**itoxantrone	Breast cancer
MMM	**m**itomycin, **m**ethotrexate, **m**itoxantrone	Breast cancer
Modified de Gramont	leucovorin, bolus fluorouracil, 46 hour infusion fluorouracil on day 1, every 14 days	Colorectal cancer
MOPP	nitrogen **m**ustard, vincristine (**O**ncovin), **p**rocarbazine, **p**rednisolone	Hodgkin's lymphoma
M-VAC	**m**ethorexate, **v**inblastine, doxorubicin (**A**driamycin), **c**isplatin	Bladder cancer
MVP	**m**itomycin, **v**inblastine, cis**p**latin	Non-small cell lung cancer and mesothelioma
PCV	**p**rocarbazine, lomustine (**C**CNU), **v**incristine	Brain tumours
PMitCEBO	**p**rednisolone, **mit**oxantrone, **c**yclophosphamide, **e**toposide, **b**leomycin, vincristine (**O**ncovin)	Non-Hodgkin's lymphoma
TAC	docetaxel (**T**axotere), doxorubicin (**A**driamycin), **c**yclophosphamide	Breast cancer
VAD	**v**incristine, doxorubicin (**A**driamycin), **D**examethasone	Multiple myeloma
VAPEC-B	**v**incristine, doxorubicin (**A**driamycin), **p**rednisolone, **e**toposide, **c**yclophosphamide, **b**leomycin	Hodgkin's lymphoma and non-Hodgkin's lymphoma

Index